Baby Steps to Better Health:
A Guided Journey in Healthier Eating

Julia Jones, MA
Lisa Jones Bromfield, RN

Copyright © 2015, all rights reserved by the authors

Printed by CreateSpace

Available from Amazon.com, other retail outlets, and Kindle

Introduction: How to Use this Book

The whole idea of this book is that taking small steps towards eating more healthfully results in steps taken towards eating more healthfully. Any gain is a good thing. Most people do not succeed in changing their entire diet or approach to food overnight. Neither of us did. We both took a long journey that included bits of awareness and bits of change. 'We' being 2 sisters, one of whom is an educator and editor and the other of whom used to be an educator and is a nurse. Our respective journeys were different but both were based in a succession of changes that have left us and our families blessed with the knowledge and the ability to eat healthfully. This book recognizes the difficulty of change and is designed to guide you on your own journey of baby steps. You can use some of our suggestions or all of our suggestions but any change towards a healthier diet is an investment in your own future, the future of your family and perhaps even a better present.

There are 15 Baby Steps represented by 15 chapters. Each chapter is arranged in sections: **Information** that might help you increase your resolve to change; **Reflection**, some questions to think about and answer (either in the companion workbook, in your own journal or notebook, or in your head); **Action** some steps to take; **Inspiration** some encouragement and inspiration to keep you going through the hard times, along with ideas for hopefully forgiving yourself your mistakes and trying again; and finally the **Expansion** section for those who want more detail on the points provided, science shared, etc. The workbook is available at our website for download or to pull up in a separate window and fill out as you read. (http://foodrealfood.com/wp-content/workbook.pdf).

If you are a woman (or man) of action and don't really want the explanations or information, then feel free to skip right to the ACTION portion of the chapter which gives you actual Baby Steps. We've presented the steps in an order that makes sense to us, but take a look at the Table of Contents and if something in particular seems like a better starting point – go for it! Any order to the steps is fine because they are all baby steps and all can contribute to goals regarding your health, how you feel, how you feed others, and/or how you look. It's your journey. We start the book with a brief look at our own journeys which we hope will amuse and encourage you to begin your own. These sections are also not 'required reading' but may be of interest to you as you discern the need for change in your own life. There are multiple beginnings to each journey and it is always nice to have companions along the way.

3.

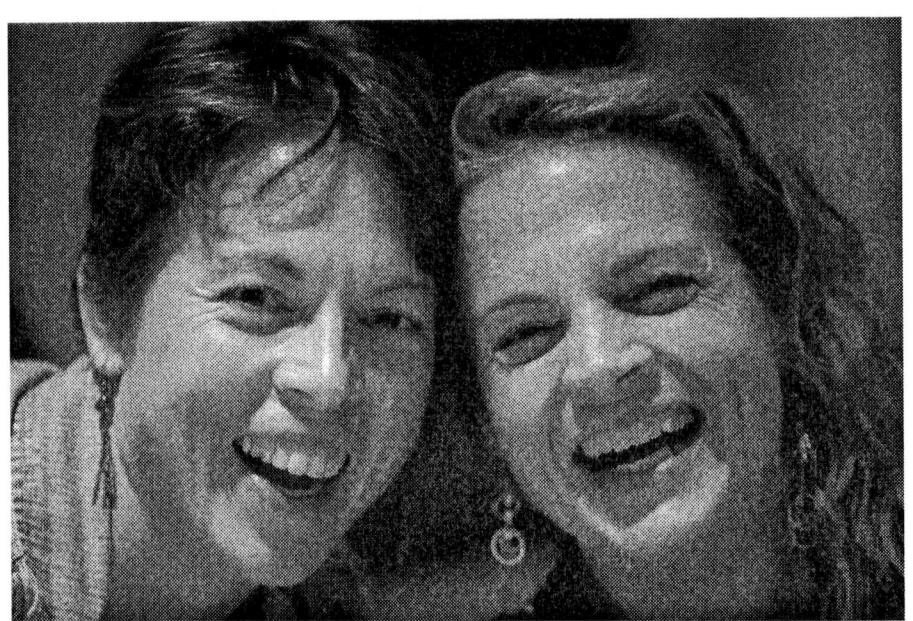

Table of Contents

Introduction: How to Use this Book 2

Why We Eat the Way We Eat 6

CHAPTER 1: Baby Step #1 13

    Action: Baby Step #1 - The Ol' Switcheroo 15

    The Top Ten Nasties 15

CHAPTER 2: Baby Step #2 22

    Action: Baby Step #2 - Be Fearless, Be Honest 23

CHAPTER 3: Baby Step #3 - Pantry Perusal 26

    Action: Baby Step #3 - Pantry Perusal 26

CHAPTER 3B: Baby Step 3B - Peeping in our Pantries 29

    Action: Pantry Preparation 33

        Short List of Easy Dinners: 34

CHAPTER 4: Baby Step 4 - Adventurousness, Experimentation and Gratitude 38

    Action: Baby Step # 4 - Acceptance and Gratitude 39

CHAPTER 5: Baby Step #5 - It's Time to Make a Plan 43

    Action: Planning Your Baby Steps 44

CHAPTER 6: Baby Step #6 - New Habits, New Rewards 54

    Action: Develop New Habits and New Rewards 56

CHAPTER 7: Baby Step 7 – Einstein's Elephant or RE-Con Convenience 59

    Action: Where does the time go? 60

CHAPTER 8: Baby Step 8 – You Deserve Real Food 66

    Action: Change your language, your mind and your habits 68

CHAPTER 9: Baby Step 9 – Bold Baby Steps, Step Up to Real Food 74

    Action: Back away from the processed foods slowly with your hands up. ... 74

CHAPTER 10: Baby Step 10 – What'll You Have? 81

    Action: Less is Less 83

CHAPTER 11: Baby Step 11 – Finding and Doling out the Food Dollars 87

    Action: Comparing the cost of healthy food / real food versus unhealthy food / processed food. 90

        Cheap Recipes 95

CHAPTER 12: Baby Step 12 – Winning at the Grocery Store 97
   Action: What to Do? A Grocery Strategy for Regular Folks 99
CHAPTER 13: Baby Step 13 – Saving on Produce 103
   Action: Shop Smart / Use Smart 103
CHAPTER 14: Baby Step 14 – Add Some Nourishment 109
   Action: Nourish Yourself 110
CHAPTER 15: Baby Step 15 – Shake Your Groove Thing 114
   Action: Easy Ways to Get Moving 117
In Conclusion 119
Recipes! 120
   Appetizers & Dips 121
   Bread Recipes 127
   Breakfast Recipes 132
   Desserts & Sweets 143
   Entrees 160
   Salad Dressing 204
   Sauces 205
   Sides 211
   Smoothies and Frozen Treats 224
   Soups 227

Why We Eat the Way We Eat

Bigg Sis: How I came to eat thoughtfully. Or in the words of Steve Martin, "Hey Kid! Don't put your lips on that[1]!"

Sleepiness, poverty, vanity, depression and motherhood improved my health. Needing to stay awake to study, not having much money for food, wanting to be thin like a movie star, feeling really low especially after eating sugar... all of these motivations provided lessons about food additives and healthy eating. Once I started gardening and became a mother, the manure really hit the fan and I achieved the status of "Food Nazi" in my family. This moniker was firmly attached to me by Biggest Bro who when I expressed dismay over the Reese's Puffs cereal in his hand one morning on vacation and foolishly stated, "You're not going to feed that to your children are you?" He replied, "Yup. And I'm going to eat some myself, Food Nazi." I knew right away that name was sticking – right in my big mouth!

Let me take you back to the beginning of my journey. Addressing how sleepiness improved my health starts off with a true confession. I was a Pepper. Way back in the earliest days of the Nutrasweet Geologic Era (it was approved for use in beverages in 1983), Diet Dr. Pepper was the manna that brought me through the wilderness of sleeplessness to study for college chemistry and paleontology. I probably drank 3-4 twelve ounce cans per day. (You can tell how old I am by the serving size). At any rate, after struggling with multiple headaches for months, someone suggested that maybe I was drinking too much caffeine. I stopped the Diet Dr. Pepper and the headaches went away. The headaches went away quickly and completely. I may have lived the rest of my life believing caffeine gives me headaches but as I was then struggling with the next year of my geology curriculum, including physics, caffeine was a necessity. I tried coffee. No headaches. Coffee merely provided blissful wakefulness to help me try to make mathematical sense of the physical universe*. Since that period of about 1 year when I consumed lots of diet soda, I would estimate that I get 2-3 headaches per year as opposed to 2-3 per day. This was the first time that I questioned the chemicals present in my food.

Next up on the list of factors that changed my eating habits... poverty. Still a college student, (turns out college is a hobby of mine) with very little money, I never ate red meat. Much cheaper to buy ramen noodles and scramble an egg into the drained noodles. I ate a lot of cheap yogurt and cheese as well. I spent a weekend at my Mother's house when she thoughtfully provided lots of my favorites such as chili with ground beef, ham and bacon. WaHoo! Fat City! Literally. I was a happy camper at first until I was having digestive problems that did not include vomiting. Enough said. Based on the probably untrue information that one temporarily loses the ability to digest red meat when not consumed regularly, I decided to stop eating it entirely. Yes, I am a bit of an extremist, but truth is that red meat was never as high on my list as carbs.

Since then, it seems to me that I probably was reacting to the sudden influx of animal fat and would have been fine in a few days. However, there is lots of evidence that our polluted, medicated, population of mammalian livestock who are forced to eat unnatural foods and to live in many inches of their own manure are not the best choice to include on our plates. So cows and pigs are out for me. The animals that I eat come from the bird and fish classes and are raised cleanly and humanely. As I have never tried reptiles or amphibians, I remain with the aforementioned categories, but if it all tastes like chicken anyway, why bother branching out? Although this incident did not provide the cut and dry cause and effect of diet soda, it was another step on the road to paying more attention to what I choose to eat.

Now we move on to the oldest and least flattering motivator. Vanity. Vanity has driven me to try and be slim and youthful: from the moment in high school in which I realized that as 'Adelaide' in *Guys and Dolls* I would have to strip down to skimpy lingerie in front of the school; to the demands of thinking a slimmer self will attract a better and more appropriate mate; to moments of examining my post childbirth, middle-aged belly. Vanity helps me eat less fat and sweets. I like to think that as an independent thinker with an appreciation of my cerebral and artistic skills I don't care so much if those jeans show my belly or not, but I do.

Over the years I tried a few diets, nothing terribly wacky except for a short foray into the cabbage soup diet, with the aim of being thinner than any of my ancestors. Of course, dieting for vanity's sake does not always lead people to increased health, but at some point I decided, "What if I just eat lots of fruits and vegetables and decrease sweets for a few weeks. Maybe that would work?" I know. I missed my calling as a rocket scientist. Key to this approach was that I only thought I'd do it for a short while, so it was not overwhelming. To be honest I was also a little depressed at the time as I was going through a divorce and felt that maybe this change in diet would also make me feel a little better. Of course I lost weight. But better than slimming down, I DID feel better. I had more energy, slept better at night, and was more in control of my emotions than prior to the change in diet. This made it a lot easier to continue to eat more fruits and vegetables and less sweets. In fact, it has been my experience that if I go long enough without a 'bad' food, say doughnuts which I love, when I do eat that food I can see the negative effect it has on how I feel. With some foods, like milk chocolate, prolonged deprivation has caused the food to entirely lose its appeal.

Currently, I once in a while deem the taste to be worth the negative effect and I eat that doughnut. But I now can eat a doughnut about once a year and be done with doughnuts for the next year. I am not at all tempted by the Hostess powdered doughnuts that show up in the employee lounge at work. They're just not good enough to be worth how they'll make me feel. I know how good I can feel when I eat right and exercise. When I don't do those things, I don't feel so good, and I miss it. Now that I am 50, I really notice it, but I was 26 when the above experiment took place, so you don't have to be my age to get signals from your body. Paying attention to my body in the form of vanity still plays a part in my choices, but I am grateful that when I make bad choices the attention paid to how I feel has resulted in the following reminder from my body, "Why are you doing that? That makes me feel like crap! And when I feel like crap I am not as likely to cooperate with all your big plans and dreams, so knock it off!" Sorry body. I am still learning.

Further interest in eating more vegetables came with growing them. I didn't backhoe the yard and plant rows and rows of vegetables. In true Baby Steps fashion, I started with 2 tomato plants in the backyard. Tomatoes can also be grown in pots on the deck or balcony. Homegrown tomatoes are a completely different taste and texture than what can be purchased at the grocery store. I think eating fresh fruits and vegetables makes you crave more fresh fruits and vegetables. Personally, I found digging, sowing and reaping to be healthy for body, mind and spirit, but most pertinent to this book, it also made me aware of all of the potential chemicals and situations used to raise the foods that I consume.

The last big personal effect came after discovering that a first time pregnancy at age 36 qualified me as AMA (advanced maternal age). That was a sunshiny moment. I decided that perhaps a 'high risk pregnancy' gal ought to eat really healthfully. Before someone tattles on me, I will confess that I stopped on the way home from my teaching job one day to purchase and consume a rather large bag of chocolate covered peanut clusters from the bulk section, yes the BULK section, and I sent my husband out on 1, maybe it was 2, occasions to "BUY ME FRENCH FRIES, NOW! (please)." But overall, I ate lean meats, fruits and vegetables, whole grains and dairy including some ice cream. I felt great once I got past the first trimester and the whole family has eaten that way ever since.

Now, after the discovery that my husband has digestive problems that preclude eating gluten or dairy, the whole family subsists on fruits, vegetables, whole grains (no gluten for hubby, less for the rest of us), and smaller amounts of fish and organic chicken. As far as feeding a child this way goes, rest assured children do get used to what you give them and although I get complaints about things my son feels are lacking in his lunch, he eats what I prepare and loves my baked goods, despite the fact that they are made with whole grain flour, other wholesome and recognizable ingredients, and far less sugar than is found in commercial products.

Lastly, I have seen the effects of healthy vs. unhealthy food on my child. My son struggled with behavior issues in pre-school. He did not throw tantrums but he had difficulty mediating his responses to other children: hugged too hard; didn't seem to understand their games all the time; at times seemed overwhelmed by noise and crowding. He did not like movie theaters. He seemed to find them too dark and close and would start asking to leave about 15 minutes into the movie. He did not peacefully sit through a kid's movie in a theater until he was just about to turn 6. It was suggested to me by several pre-school teachers that perhaps he had a sensory integration disorder and I should have him tested.

I was a special ed teacher for a few years and this didn't ring true for me. He is very bright and sensitive such that he could not watch any violence or frightening material, or even intensely joyful movies until he was about 9. Even then we were, and remain, careful about what he watches. I did not have him tested because I saw different behaviors in different places and felt that he was finding ways to deal with his sensitivity and his unique brain. I did notice however, that it was extremely difficult for him to exhibit good behavior when he ate lots of sugar, or white flour products, i.e. simple carbohydrates. My mother was dubious about the connection, although she kindly kept that to herself until one night in a very slow restaurant. My son was very hungry and I foolishly did not have any healthy snacks with me. I let him have the cracker bowl and as my Mom and Little Sis and I chatted, he went through about ten 2 packs of saltine crackers. Shortly after dinner (which he didn't eat much of being full of simple carbs, i.e. sugar) he melted down entirely. My mother looked amazed and said, "You were right!" And I was right. I saw the same problems with my 'ADHD' special ed students as well. Regardless of what doctors and researchers may say about the causes of, cures for, or reality of, ADHD, I will tell you that it makes an ADHD student's job at school much tougher if he or she starts the day off with a can of sweetened beverage and a pastry.

Feeding myself and my family healthfully has been a long journey of discovery, success and flops. The flops were never failures because we still had something to eat and let's face it, convenience foods are not always that great either. The changes have happened gradually, one baby step at a time. It is my sincere hope that boiling down this long experiment and all of these degrees of change will assist you in your own quest for increased health for you and your family, whether you be driven by sleepiness, financial troubles, health problems, vanity or advanced maternal age!

* Coffee later proved to be too much of a stimulant for me as in my late 20's it began to cause rapid and irregular heartbeats. The withdrawal of coffee identified the culprit and to this day I cannot consume large amounts of caffeine or I have the same problems. Thankfully, a bit of dark chocolate is not an issue! Yet again, a health problem caused and solved by what I consume.

Little Sis: How I came to eat thoughtfully. Or how I learned to appreciate hi test fuel.

I have a vivid memory of a food shopping trip from my tween years. My parents had separated and my father and I went to the store together. THIS was not a good shopping crew. We came home excited with our bounty. Little Debbies for lunches, chocolate chip cookies, ice cream and lots of other goodies. I have no idea if this was intended to be an actual grocery run, but I DO remember my sister's reaction to our haul: "Guys. Where's the food? Where's the rest of it?"

My sister hadn't even begun her transformation yet, but she already knew that packaged sweets do not a meal make, and this is because we grew up on homemade food. While it wasn't necessarily what I would choose now, and I'm sure I did my fair share of grousing, for the most part we ate at home, with indications from our parents as to what part of the plate was required eating, and with food that had been cooked rather than assembled. I think this was a pretty solid foundation for potentially healthy eating.

My problems with food really kicked into gear as an adolescent when I really wanted to change my body shape. I wanted to be a little pixie person; genetics be damned. As supervision of my actual intake decreased through my teen years I embarked on a journey of bizarre and poor food choices that likely worsened my situation. For breakfast – giant bowl of high fiber cereal. For lunch – a grapefruit or giant apple and a diet coke. For dinner – entirely dependent on whether or not there was play practice that night. If so, I would often eat carry out with friends as rehearsal time didn't really match up with go home and eat dinner time. If no practice, I would sometimes make myself a giant bowl of frozen vegetables or make some pasta. What's wrong with this picture? It left a lot of hunger that usually got filled with crap. When you get really hungry, it's awfully hard not to eat crap when it's offered or available. When you're an adolescent and potentially not in your right mind at any given moment, there's no governor of portion or ingredients. My part time jobs were mostly in food establishments and I was more than happy to take care of mistake sundaes or oops fries. I had pretty much left the realm of reasonable and routine eating.

College helped in that there was this regularly scheduled opportunity to eat with other people who were also eating, but the siren call of that cereal bar full of all the cereals that had never been available at home was pretty loud. My alma mater is also blessed with an onsite dairy that provided the ice cream for the dining hall. Oh mercy. If it's not enough to eat it, you can put it in your coffee you know. That'll fuel some late night study.

The years proceeded and as the jobs of my twenties flew by I learned to cook enough to get by. It wasn't until my second year of teaching that Mr. Little Sis and I looked at each other (and our increasing girth) and decided we might need to make some changes. Bigg Sis was already many baby steps down the road to healthier eating, and with good knowledge of our culinary preferences, she made a very sound suggestion. "What if you just switched out regular pasta for whole grain pasta? What if you just tried to do that one thing?" I think I ignored the first and perhaps second iteration of that suggestion, but the first-year-teacher consolation Cherry Garcia ice cream eating had made it patently obvious that some change would be required. And so we made that one switch. Frankly, we found that we liked whole grain pasta better. We felt more satisfied after eating. This change trickled into other changes: whole grain bread, less junk food, more real food. We experimented with Weight Watchers and were both very successful, discovering that the point systems they use (if you don't just decide to eat a sundae and skip food the rest of the day) really do lead you to the conclusion that more vegetables and whole grains are good steps to take.

While these changes were taking place Mr. Big Sis had a job that required us to travel to Northern California a few times a year. It wasn't long before our journey to real food included a wonderful excursion into foodie land. There are so many reasons to give up junk food in foodie land. We really enjoyed foodie land, and still do when we ever so occasionally have the opportunity to be really picky about the provenance of our olives. Reality, however, when it comes, can be quite jarring.

Nothing is so jarring a reality as being new parents, except being new parents of more than one infant. Our twins rocked our world. The months leading up to their arrival and their infancy really deepened our sense that the grocery store was filled with food we didn't want to eat or feed our children. That sense has grown over the years and turned from a negative sense of all the junk that is out there to eat into a positive sense of all the wonderful real and healthful food that is also out there, even if it is at times harder to find. My recent forays into forgoing meat and dairy (dairy being an avoid all the time food and meat an avoid most of the time food) were largely a result of the series of food related documentaries that have come out in the last 10 years. I was slowly convinced that perhaps cutting animal products was worth a try.

For me personally, and I've come to believe that from a body perspective this result is INDEED very personal, going without dairy is a game changer. My seasonal allergies have diminished to the point that they are only an occasional annoyance (a revolution from a lifetime of medication and tissues). When I really pay attention, it is much easier to lose weight than it has been in the past. I rarely have stomach troubles or reflux or anything like that. The whole system seems to work better. So all of my experiments have led me slowly to a place where I don't eat dairy, I only sometimes eat meat and the rest of what is on my plate is generally something that is grown from a plant. And I feel great.

It is the "I feel great" part that really makes all this baby stepping, experimenting, and learning worthwhile. While I can't say that I am in a permanent state of perfect health (I have school aged children and am therefore doomed to some continual level of viral sharing), I feel better than I ever have. I have more energy. I feel more fit. I can breathe better. It also seems that when I do get sick, it doesn't tend to stick around as long. I've not been part of a study and I'm not a scientist, but I'm pretty comfortable concluding that a good bit of this has to do with the way that I feed my body. And knowing that I can have that impact with the choices I make sure does make it easier to keep up the good work, to keep making good choices, and to catch myself when I fall.

CHAPTER 1: Baby Step #1: The Ol' Switcheroo: Finding New Favorites, One Change at a Time

INFORMATION:

We have too much information about food extremes and not enough about what is readily available to us.

When it comes to sharing information about food, and about most things, the media has two tents. They occupy a very large tent at the negative end of the spectrum and a very small tent at the positive end of the spectrum. Both ends are spectacular and intense and sell news. But most of us live our lives in the middle. Sure we've heard about the super foods AND we've heard about the recalls of food due to bacterial outbreaks or the latest extreme food scare. Then there are the periodic scares that are reversed, like the dangers of caffeine- no caffeine is not bad.... Well it IS bad, but not so bad, but it's not really bad at all. In the same article from US News & World Report, (Shute, 2007)[2] readers are given both sides of the story in that caffeine has been found to reduce the risk of Parkinson's disease, decrease migraines and due to its antioxidant content, reduce risk of colon cancer, gallstones, and liver cancer. Simultaneously, caffeine can cause stomach pain and gastrointestinal reflux, anxiety and heart palpitations in the caffeine sensitive, and may decrease ability to get pregnant while possibly increasing risk of miscarriage and of having a low weight birth baby. How's a person to decide what to eat anymore?

Moderation is of course one answer, especially to the question of something like caffeine, but we can also eat the foods in the middle of the spectrum - with a smattering of the outrageous, special or ridiculously expensive foods when we have the ability or desire! There exists an abundance of regular food that is surprisingly delicious, healthy and easy to prepare. Unfortunately we are also confronted with way too much 'regular' food, or what has become regular food, that is surprisingly dangerous to our health. Let's take a look at the middle – at the blueberries, brown rice, lentils and hummus as opposed to the latest of the expensive healthy food trends which get so much attention in the positive media tent. Likewise, the media gives the negative extremes enough attention, let's focus on sugar and the chemical soup of processed foods rather than on *e. coli*, listeria and the latest scare.

Finding the wholesome, good food and getting off of the bad food-like-stuff is the theme of Baby Step #1. Our experience is that this is most effectively done in stages or steps. Although there are a few individuals out there who can successfully change their entire diet all at once, those individuals are very rare and generally avoided by the rest of us ;-). Food has a lot of importance in our lives because it fills more than just a nutritional function. Therefore it is wise to move slowly, with reflection, and make sure we aren't setting ourselves up for failure by changing everything at once. We are not suggesting that you give up all your favorite tastes, comforts and conveniences. We are suggesting that you make a change in your diet and your approach to eating by swapping an unhealthy food for a healthy or healthier food.

REFLECTION: *Change is not an all or nothing process.*

Easing the progress of any change is the confidence that you can handle change. You CAN handle the truth, right? Unfortunately, for most of us, part of any change is remembering the times we failed to complete a previously attempted change. We all fail and we all sabotage future success by focusing, highlighting, dwelling on, gnawing on, and losing sleep over, our failures.

> *1a) Have you ever tried to change your eating habits before?*
>
> *1b) How did it go?*
>
> *1c) What happened?*
>
> *1d) How did it make you feel?*
>
> *(Available in <u>Workbook</u>)*

One reason the Sis sisters came up with our Baby Steps plan was to provide do-able changes that will not only reward you with the outcome of the change, but will provide you with a success. And it doesn't need to be a total smashing success, because food choices are not permanent. We have many opportunities to get it right, everyday. And remember:

This is not a test of your character.
This is not a one-time opportunity.
This is not an indication of your ability to lead a meaningful life.
This is a choice, a choice that you get to make several times a day.

Don't you love do-overs?

I once took a class on parenting that offered some wonderful solutions to discipline that work best when delivered by a sane, rational adult who has had enough sleep. Yeah, right, I haven't met many of those. But the teacher left us with a profound message. "If you do it this way more than 50% of the time, you are doing a great job as a parent[3]." I found that to be very helpful and I think it is relevant here as well. Parenting and eating are very similar in that we do them a lot, and have lots of tries to do it differently. It is better to do the right thing some of the time than none of the time, and really great to do the right thing most of the time!

> *1e) How you would respond to a friend who was trying to make a change like getting more exercise by adding one walk a week – would you encourage or scold?*
>
> *1f) Can you be as kind and encouraging to yourself?*

Baby Steps to Better Health / Baby Step #1   15.

(Available in Workbook)

Enough chopping and dicing, let's put the goods in the frying pan!

ACTION: Baby Step #1 - The Ol' Switcheroo

Switch out some nasty thing from your diet and replace it with something healthier. One item. One switch. As often as possible.

If you are having trouble choosing, below are our suggestions. You might consider this a master list to work through over time, one item at a time.

As you read on, and before you finalize your choice of what you are going to swap out, consider the function of that item in your life. Is this an item that provides energy or alertness? (mocha latte, sugar), an item that provides comfort, an item that is part of your routine, an item of convenience, a tradition, a reward? Knowing the function of this food will help you successfully replace that food with something that fulfills the same function. For example, if you are not looking to replace caffeine but are wanting to make a low sugar switch for your morning Coke, then you should replace the caffeine portion of the Coke with tea or coffee (that has less sugar than Coke... or no sugar at all) or you will be hurting for your caffeine and probably not stick to your plan.

> *1g) What item could you give up that would make you feel better about yourself?*
>
> *1h) Is it something you know you shouldn't be eating?*
>
> *1i) Is it something that is eating into your budget?*
>
> *1j) Is it something that you feel you can give up so you can start with a success?*
>
> *(Available in Workbook)*

THE TOP TEN NASTIES. Choose one. Lose one. Refuse one. You'll be glad you did!

There is more info in the Expansion section at the end of this chapter on what makes these things so very nasty. Underlined recipes are found at the page in parentheses after the recipe.

1) Soda / sweetened beverages (energy drinks, juice cocktails & sport drinks)

Replace with:
- water (it's the original drink you know!!),

Baby Steps to Better Health / Baby Step #1

- water and 50% soda or juice to help you cut back,
- water and lemon or lime,
- iced tea (with less sugar than soda. You can slowly reduce the sugar in your tea over time as well),
- coffee (unless you have heart issues – then check with your MD),
- a smaller quantity of soda: drink half as much, then half again as much - just work your way towards as little soda as possible,
- homemade Sports Drink that is MUCH less sweet .

2) Doritos / Cheetos / Potato chips – especially flavored ones (lots of nasty chemicals).

Replace with:
- homemade popcorn,
- healthy crackers with very short ingredient lists that include whole grains (i.e. Triscuits),
- kale chips,
- crunchy veggies dipped in hummus(p123) or salsa or sunflower cheese(p122),
- small serving of nuts (watch the salt if your MD tells you to do so).
- If you need a teeny baby step on this one, switch from flavored to plain chips.

3) Commercially pre-made baked goods like donuts, cookies, cakes, lunchbox treats

Replace with:
- homemade baked goods (see Desserts and Sweets section, p143),
- peanut butter and jelly on whole wheat bread,
- flavored herb tea,
- a small serving of dark chocolate,
- a healthy cracker or whole grain bread with some dark chocolate (very nice together),
- a bit of Chocolate Almond Butter(p134) on a carrot or healthy cracker or bread,
- a piece of fruit.

4) Fake dairy like Cool whip, Hazelnut flavored goo (I mean fake-coffee-creamer-stuff), powdered coffee creamer, i.e. all of those evil oil-based imposters for anything edible.

Replace with:
- a little REAL dairy or if you don't do dairy try a nut or coconut based milk, small amount of sugar and maybe a drop or two of vanilla or some cinnamon in your coffee, (make a batch of this to last for a few days),
- Date Cream(p135)
- flavored coffee with cream (the flavor is in the roasted beans –probably mostly chemicals but a step in the right direction)

5) Boxed macaroni & cheese (includes Hamburger Helper type stuff)

Replace with:
- real recipes for fast versions of these dishes that use wholesome ingredients and no chemicals,
- fast, easy version of homemade macaroni & cheese(p174),

Baby Steps to Better Health / Baby Step #1 17.

- add cooked fresh or frozen veggies and shredded cheese to pasta,
- microwave potatoes and top with some shredded cheese and/or salsa and cooked veggies.

We are halfway through the list…HANG IN THERE! You don't have to make changes for everything on this list. You are reading the list to choose <u>one</u> switch. Keep reading, or if it's overwhelming or depressing, choose something out of the first 5. The switch is for you… to improve your health and the way you care for yourself.

6) Candy (high quality dark chocolate in reasonable quantities is another story).

Replace with:
- homemade treats in reasonable quantity,
- small serving of dark chocolate (1 – 2 oz.),
- flavored herbal tea,
- brushing your teeth – (sometimes the mint flavor takes away the craving for something sweet),
- if you eat a lot of candy and drink a lot of soda, you are probably addicted to sugar, so set a reasonable goal of reducing how much you eat. Keep lowering your amount, and re-choose when and if you slip.

7) Commercial salad dressing. Ewwwww – read the label, seriously.

Replace with:
- homemade dressings(p204), some of which are incredibly simple,
- olive, walnut, avocado or grapeseed oil and vinegar of your choice splashed right on top,
- avocado pieces in the salad and a drizzle of vinegar.

8) White crackers & flavored crackers with more than 5 ingredients. Read the labels of your crackers.

Replace with:
- short wholesome ingredient list crackers (Triscuits ingredient list = wheat, oil and salt),
- dip a healthier cracker into salsa, or add real cheese or plant based cheese like Little Sis' sunflower cheese(p122) or hummus(p124).
See chips substitutes (#2) for more ideas.

9) Fast Food.

Replace with:
- salad bar or hot food prepared at a grocery store,
- pack leftovers for lunch when cleaning up the evening meal (you may want to start making more at dinner just to accommodate lunches).
- Investigate the somewhat healthier fast food choices as an interim such as Subway or Panera bread,
- Whole grain pasta and sauce with a salad.
If you are eating a lot of fast food, commit to eat at home or pack a lunch one or more

times per week when you would have eaten fast food.
If you haven't seen it yet, I recommend watching the documentary *Super Size Me* with your family (watch first to assess the appropriateness, there is some frank talk about sex, but nothing graphic, and a bit of bad language).

10) Commercial white bread (and even some 'whole wheat' bread); read the labels.

Replace with:
- whole wheat breads that list whole wheat flour before listing white flour (make sure you read the labels).
- sandwiches using romaine lettuce leaves instead of bread (A homemade lettuce wrap - healthy and sophisticated… Hey Now!)
- brown rice, quinoa, millet, or barley as a side dish instead of bread

Wrapping up the Action: Baby Steps for Baby Step #1

1-1) Think of (write down if you like) some candidates for switching

1-2) Decide what you would replace them with

1-3) Acknowledge the function of each item

1-4) Choose one to start with

1-5) Choose a period of time that you will make this switch for.

> Jeremy Dean is a psychologist who also suggests breaking the process of changing habits into small pieces. In his book, *Making Habits Breaking Habits: How to Make Changes That Stick*[4], he states that it is better to replace a habit than to simply be rid of it and that it can take 21 days to establish a new simple habit. The Sis sisters have also heard 2 weeks and 30 days as periods of time that can help establish a new habit.

1-6) At the end of that time assess how it went and see if you can commit to lengthening the time and perhaps adding a second swap into your food life.

(Available in Workbook)

INSPIRATION:

Be realistic and remember a permanent Baby Step is further along than a Giant Step with a Giant retreat.

Set your sights on an achievable goal. If you think you can only cut your consumption of one of the above in half, then make that decision and set a goal of 2 weeks. At the end of the 2 weeks commit again and decide if you can cut back some more. If you slip,

Baby Steps to Better Health / Baby Step #1

if you slide, if you make a poor choice, it is not a permanent fail. Your chooser is not broken, it's just not perfect. If it was perfect, you probably would have already been recalled to the place where perfect humans go. You are still a wonderful human being with potential for joy, love, productivity, creativity and health. Just decide to try and make a different choice the next time and keep on the road to better health, one baby step at a time. Remember:

> This is not a test of your character.
>
> This is not a one-time opportunity.
>
> This is not an indication of your ability to lead a meaningful life.
>
> This is a choice that you get to make several times a day.

EXPANSION: *More info about the top 10 nasties*

Some people find it motivating to know the nitty gritty of why these foods are unhealthy. Others don't want to be bogged down in the details. Feel free to read or move on to the next chapter, when you're ready!

1) Soda.
A 12 oz serving of Coca Cola has 39 grams of sugar which is about 9.5 teaspoons. A regular sized Snicker's bar has 30 grams of sugar or about 7.5 teaspoon of sugar[5]. Can you imagine putting 9 teaspoons of sugar on your cereal or in your iced tea? That's a lot of sugar.

Most sodas are sweetened primarily with high fructose corn syrup (HFCS). Despite the corn industry's attempts to state that their product is not harmful, the Center for Science in the Public Interest (CSPI) reports that "large amounts (of HFCS) promote tooth decay, as well as increase triglyceride (fat) levels in blood, thereby increasing the risk of heart disease. There is evidence that HFCS may promote fatty liver disease, insulin resistance (which leads to Type 2 Diabetes), increased abdominal fat (which leads to metabolic syndrome) and decreased ability to trigger hormones that tell you when you are full[6]. The HFCS that is used in most soft drinks contains about 10 percent more fructose than sucrose. That makes most soft drinks a bit more harmful than if they were made with sugar" (CSPI, 2012).

According to the children's health section of WebMD, "Nearly 90 studies have linked sweetened beverages and children's weight problems. Even one or two sweet drinks a day can cause a problem[7]." Higher childhood obesity rates have caused higher rates of 'adult' diseases in children such as type II diabetes, high blood pressure, high cholesterol and high tri-glycerides. All of these diseases increase the risk for heart disease and stroke. According to the American Heart Association, obesity negatively affects every system in the body and is more detrimental to health than smoking or excessive drinking[8].

Baby Steps to Better Health / Baby Step #1

2) Doritos / Cheetos /Potato chips – especially flavored ones (lots of nasty chemicals). Chips like these contain lots of fat and ingredients like the following from the ingredient list for nacho cheese Doritos (from the Doritos website on 8/11/13)[9] Yellow 6, Yellow 5 (both of which are on the Center for Science in the Public Interest's list of food additives[10] to avoid), Red 40 (which is on the CSPI's caution list), MSG (which is on the CSPI's list of causing problems for some people), and artificial flavor (which I can't condemn or condone because we don't know what it is) – and a huge amount of sodium. While the CSPI does not consider MSG to be anything more than an allergen for some people, there are many researchers who disagree and claim that MSG is addictive and causes many health problems including migraines[11].

3) Pre-made baked goods like donuts, cookies, cakes, lunchbox treats
Read your labels. You will usually find no whole grain flour and lots of chemicals (including azidocarbamide with which you can also clean your boat). Look for and avoid baked goods that contain the following per the Food Additive list from CSPI[8]:

AVOID	CAUTION	CUT BACK
Caramel coloring	Sucralose	Corn syrup
Partially hydrogenated vegetable oil		Salatrim (manufactured fat)
Hydrogenated vegetable oil		Dextrose (sugar)
Potassium bromate (banned everywhere in world except Japan and US)		sucrose
Saccharin		

You can find detailed information about these ingredients at the CSPI website[12]. Michael Pollan, author of *The Omnivore's Dilemma* suggests that you not purchase anything that contains more than 5 ingredients. I would add to that by saying that if you don't know what it is, and don't know where it came from… don't eat it.

4) Fake dairy like Cool whip, Hazelnut flavored goo (I mean coffee creamer stuff), powdered coffee creamer, etc. – those oil-based imposters for anything edible. Here is a list of ingredients for Coffee Mate hazelnut powdered creamer: Sugar, vegetable oil (partially hydrogenated coconut or palm kernel, hydrogenated soybean), corn syrup solids, sodium caseinate (a milk derivative), and less than 2% of dipotassium phosphate (moderates coffee acidity), mono- and diglycerides (prevents oil separation), sodium aluminosilicate, salt, natural and artificial flavor. Partially hydrogenated oils are trans fats. They are on the AVOID list of the CSPI. And if that's not enough to

Baby Steps to Better Health / Baby Step #1

dissuade you, just say 'corn syrup solids' 10 times fast and see if you still want to consume them.

5) Boxed macaroni & cheese (This includes Hamburger Helper type stuff)
Most of these have artificial colors in them, PLUS much less nutritional value than what you could make at home. MSG is in almost all processed foods, so again, although there is disagreement about what if anything other than allergies, can be caused by MSG, I do not plan to be one of the test subjects in that food industry experiment.

6) Candy (high quality dark chocolate in reasonable quantities is another story).
It's the sugar….. and LOTS of artificial colors. Artificial colors in children's foods are banned in Europe due to the links to hyperactivity and cancer. Artificial colors are on the short list of additives that the CSPI most strongly urges people to avoid. In addition to the lousy ingredients there is the problem of empty calories. Candy has nothing to offer but a sugar high, rotten teeth, increased weight and the myriad of problems that accompany obesity.

7) Commercial salad dressing.
Lousy fats, thickeners, lots of sugar and all manner of unrecognizable items. Where's the food? Truly, you can get used to homemade dressing – make a big bottle once you find a recipe you like so you'll have it for a while! If you have 2 different recipes you like, use 2 jars to offer the variety we are so used to on the salad dressing aisle.

8) White crackers & flavored crackers with more than 5 ingredients.
Just like baked goods – lots of unnecessary and dangerous ingredients and not much nutrition.

9) Fast Food.
Sugar, fat and salt. Sugar, fat and salt. Sugar, fat and salt. Oh and don't forget the aziodocarbamide (boat cleaner) and nitrates / nitrites (cancer causing meat preservatives and on CSPI's avoid list) and 22 ingredients in the bun for a Burger King cheeseburger. Who needs 22 ingredients in a bun?

10) Commercial white bread (and even some 'whole wheat' bread)
This is a bit of a repeat of the baked goods category, but white bread is so common that it's worth a little more info. Bread manufacturers write lots of nice things on their labels to convince you of the health benefits of their products. However, the proof is in the label. It is near impossible to find a loaf of bread with 5 ingredients, but if you read labels before buying you can limit the nasties while improving the nutrition by ensuring the presence of whole grain, fiber, and protein.

CHAPTER 2: Baby Step #2: An Honest Look at What You Eat Now

INFORMATION: *Diets don't work.*

The diet industry is a multi-billion dollar industry full of failure. How do they keep on raking in the dough? We all know that most weight loss programs are NOT losing propositions – weight might be lost for a while, but it usually returns. If we ourselves haven't tried diets and failed, then we know lots of people who have. It is not easy to lose weight in our society. We don't exercise enough and we eat too much. But is it just eating too much? There is a lot of research showing that certain foods (processed foods that are high in sugar, salt and unhealthy fat) make us crave more of the very things which are bad for our health[13]. Although I can't prove it, it seems to me that the reason we're still hungry after that bag of chips is quite simple. Our bodies know when they've been had. They know when they've chewed up a bunch of stuff that is really not that good for them and they still crave some nutrition. But we, having been blinded, tempted and trained to seek out the Ka-Pow of high sugar, salt and fat just go for more of that sugar, salt, and fat. Change what you eat and you will not only change your body, but you will change what you crave and how you feel about food. It takes time to retrain your taste buds and your cravings, but one positive healthy change can be built on, one baby step at a time.

REFLECTION: *Deprivation doesn't motivate. Abundance motivates.*

The Sis sisters want you to feel good, to eat well, and to enjoy your food. We do not want you to go on a diet. There are so many diets out there, so many plans that will tell you exactly what you will eat and will give you a variety of ways of measuring, quantifying, and analyzing your food so that you can be sure you're staying on plan. This is not what we're about.

Baby Steps to Better Health is a way to learn how to eat real, healthful food; to learn how to change your relationship with food; and to move from a place of deprivation to a place of healthful and satisfying abundance. Baby Step #1 asked you to make a switch. We asked you to find one unhealthy item in your diet and switch it out for something healthier. Didn't do it yet? Didn't go so well? Went great? It's all good. You can jump in where we are, start from the first step, whatever you like. Any step you take towards healthier eating is a good one. Today, we're going to get started on Step 2: Be Fearless. Be Honest. Huh?

I used to teach and one of the things my colleagues and I constantly reminded ourselves was that you have to teach where the student is. You have to figure out what they know if you want to teach them something new. The same is true for any habit or change that we are trying to make, isn't it? If I want to build a table, I need to get real honest with myself about my carpentry skills; I have to see if I have the materials required; I (this is certainly true for me) would have to learn some very specific skills; then I would be ready to start building successfully, rather than making the kind of table I would make if I just started banging away with hammer and nails (and believe me I speak from experience here as I am a long-time bang away at the unknown kind of gal).

The next few baby steps are prep work, getting honest with ourselves about what we eat, investigating the materials we have on hand, and learning some new skills. Rather than thrashing about and banging away at our food, our self-esteem, our bodies, and our nerves, it seems wise to take some time to gather our resources and figure out exactly where this road starts so we can get on with making it go somewhere healthy and delicious.

ACTION: Baby Step #2 - Be Fearless, Be Honest

What I'm going to suggest here may put some of you off, and perhaps that's why I've been jabbering (stalling) here. I want to suggest that you keep a food journal… NONONONONO don't stop reading! I'm not talking about THAT kind of food journal. I don't want you to measure your stuff and write down how many calories are in things. I don't want you to assign numbers to your food. I don't want you to categorize your food and check things off. I don't want you to freak out about writing these things down.

I just want to suggest that you make a note of what you're eating (including snacks). Why? So we can have a meeting and feel bad? Not at all. The Sis sisters both know from experience that a lot of eating is driven by habit and convenience. A great deal of our munching is not really considered: it may be reflex, it may be habit, it may be a lot of things, but getting it on a piece of paper makes it really easy to look at our choices and find some places to begin, to set some goals for ourselves, to identify good candidates for the kinds of switches that we've suggested in Baby Step 1.

Be Fearless. Be Honest. Write It Down.

A few months ago I realized that I was putting on a little weight and was feeling a bit lethargic, weighed down, a little slow and unmotivated. I began to pay attention to, and to write down, what I was eating. I realized that every day while I was making dinner, there was quite a bit of snacking going on. The exact contents varied, but more often than not a fair amount of salt and fat worked their way in there. Some days I nibbled so much that I wasn't even hungry for the delicious, healthful meal I had prepared for my family. It took my attention to identify that habit, to realize that I was letting myself get too hungry at that hour and to be sure to listen to the call of the wild stomach before I became a ravening beast. I needed to see it to make the change. Once I saw it, it was very easy to identify some changes that I could make. I didn't need anybody to tell me what to cut first – I knew it. I could see it right there on the page.

Be Fearless. Be Honest. Write It Down.

So what should this food journal look like? Well, let me tell you. I don't care what it looks like. I don't care what you write it on. I don't care if you use shorthand. I don't

Baby Steps to Better Health / Baby Step #2

care if you write it with a crayon with your toes. My only recommendation is that you put it together in such a way that you will be able to look at a whole week or so without a lot of effort – so writing each day on the back of a receipt that is in your wallet full of receipts from the last 4 months (is this just me?) is probably not the way to go. Beyond that, knock yourself out. Write it wherever, however; this is YOUR exercise. You are finding the real starting point for YOUR road to healthier eating. No numbers, no measuring, just a log of what you are doing. No judgment, no fear, no recrimination. You can do this. Just take a step, with a pen (or a crayon) and a piece of paper. We want you to move from a place of deprivation to a place of healthful and satisfying abundance. You and your family deserve a place of satisfying abundance. You'll be in good company! Okay, GO!

Wrapping up the ACTION: Baby Steps for Baby Step #2:

2-1) Decide on what and where you will log this information.

2-2) Decide how long you will do this (3 days? 5 days? 1 week?).

2-3) Make an appointment with yourself (and your spouse or family if they are taking this journey with you – or maybe you will be the leader and they don't need to know yet) to review what you have recorded.

2-4) Do it!

2-5) Reward yourself with a non-food reward. If you can, choose something with increments (like time reading a novel, or how many minutes someone in the family will massage your neck) so that you can reward yourself for getting some of it done. If you don't get it all done, reward yourself for getting some of it done.

2-6) Set new goals, (to re-try recording what you eat) or to help you make more choices for swapping and trying new things that are healthier than the old things (old things does not include slightly used spouses, siblings or friends).

(Available in Workbook)

EXPANSION:

The food journal is a way to identify places for change.

As you assess what is being eaten and when, you will likely find the changes you need to make and at the very least you will identify the times when you are mind-lessly, thought-lessly eating. (We do it too!) If buying a special journal or notebook would motivate you, then do it, but it doesn't have to be fancy, just something you can read from.

Use the food journal to make note of:

Baby Steps to Better Health / Baby Step #2

A) How you feel (both physically and emotionally) after eating certain foods. Pay attention to how you are feeling and record what you ate and how you feel, good or bad!

B) How you are feeling (both physically and emotionally) when you reach for snack food.

C) Whether you are feeling poorly at the same time every day. What are you eating prior to this period?

D) How you talk yourself into (or out of) what you eat.

The information in your food journal can help you develop a list of foods that make you feel good and a list of foods that make you feel bad. Post these lists somewhere that will be visible when making choices about food. Personally, it was only noticing how badly I felt after eating doughnuts that defeated my doughnut desire (Oooh that dastardly doughnut desire). I am now able to forego the doughnuts that frequently appear in the break room at work because I KNOW I will feel badly after eating one. That is more powerful to me than worrying that I might gain some weight, or that my future health might suffer from that choice. And you may think that you will feel good after eating something that you know is really bad for you, but do you?

Finally, your food journal friend can also be a place to record your successes!

A) Make sure you record the meals or dishes that you and or your family enjoy.

B) Write a congratulatory note when you make a healthful choice.

C) Re-read success notes when you need some inspiration.

D) Reflect on changes you notice in your health, both emotional and physical as you take baby steps down the road to better health.

If you would like to, you can use space at the end of the workbook we refer to throughout the chapters.

CHAPTER 3: Baby Step #3 - What's in Your Pantry?

INFORMATION: You eat what you have.

There are many reasons, both sensible and reprehensible, why the American diet is full of chemicals and other substances that seem to wreak havoc on our bodies. Whatever the reasons, however, the result is the same – vastly increased rates of obesity, diabetes, coronary artery disease and hypertension. So what are we going to do about it? Make the change toward real food one step at a time including what we have in our pantries, in our refrigerators, or hidden in the back of the closet.

REFLECTION: We must provide ourselves with the tools to make change happen.

Even a baby step moves you forward. Look down and gaze at those lovely toes of yours and see how they are inching down the road to better health. Even a little healthier is better than no healthier… and it's a whole lot better than less healthy. In Baby Step #1 we encouraged you to swap something unhealthy for something healthier. In Baby Step #2 we suggested you keep a food journal so that you can become more aware of what you are eating. Of course you know what you are putting into your mouth, but when you think a little bit more about it, you might acknowledge places where a little more forethought and change is needed. Again – moving forward, even a little bit, makes you healthier.

If a healthful meal happens one more time a week than it used to, then you are making progress. I certainly did not change the way I feed my family dinner every night of the week in one fell swoop! (What the heck IS a swoop, anyhow?) Baby Step #3 takes you into your pantry (or cupboard, and fridge/freezer) for some more observations which may help you more easily include healthier food in your life.

A fundamental task in preparing healthful food is perusing recipes and menu ideas and adding the necessary items to your grocery list. You can't cook real food if the ingredients aren't there. The Sis sisters combat missing ingredients problems in 2 ways. First, we keep our pantries stocked with staples that can contribute to many healthy meals. Second, we are more than happy to make substitutions when we are missing an ingredient to a recipe.

ACTION: Baby Step #3 What's in Your Pantry?

Pantry perusal is taking a good look at what you keep on hand. Little Sis and I both have a short list of items that we try to always have in the pantry because they are 'go to' items. They are items that help us on the nights when there is no time, or there was no planning, or when the alternative is overpaying for some food that is bad for us.

Make a list of what's in your pantry and ask yourself the following questions:

Baby Steps to Better Health / Baby Step #3

3a) What's in your pantry; Is there food in that there food?

3b) Are the items in your pantry INGREDIENTS or are they things you need to warm up or simply unwrap to eat?

3c) Are you buying foods that you know you shouldn't eat but can't resist eating if they are in your house?

3d) Are you buying foods you would like to limit for your children?

3e) Are you buying convenience foods that are not really good, but "who has time to make that from scratch?" We're going to help you with this one... I promise!

(Available in Workbook)

Perhaps your pantry perusal brings you back to Baby Step #1 where you decided to switch something out. Maybe you're ready to make another switch like brown rice in place of instant potatoes or stuffing. Maybe you're going to replace candy with dried fruit and nuts. Maybe you're going to try some new grains like quinoa that are healthy and quick.

We are going to share our lists for what the 'go to' items are in our pantries and provide you with ideas for easy healthy meals in the next chapter. For now, here are some steps for you to take:

Wrapping up the ACTION: Baby Steps for Baby Step #3

3-1) Decide when you are going to peruse your pantry (allowing 10 – 40 minutes, whatever you can spare).

3-2) Copy the questions down or use our worksheet or skip writing all together but be prepared to make physical or mental note of what you find.

3-3) Sit down and review what you find. This will make you more aware of what kind of food is consistently present in your house.

3-4) Think of a few items that would give you more healthy options and add them to your grocery list. (If you can't think of anything, we will cover this in more depth in the next chapter).

(Available in Workbook)

Again, Baby Steps 2 & 3 are prep work. You are preparing to be enlightened (in more ways than one, know what I'm saying?). You are going to become more conscious of,

Baby Steps to Better Health / Baby Step #3

and thoughtful about, your food choices, because they are choices. They are often difficult choices, especially in light of the speed of our culture and the incredible advertising machine that profits the Prepared Foods industry at the cost of our health. Despite these obstacles, you can set yourself up for better choices if the stuff of better choices is readily available. The wonderful thing about choices regarding food is that you get another chance at the food choices at least 3 times a day.

EXPANSION: Cooking Whole Grains

Alternative grains are a staple in the Sis sister's pantries because they can be the underpinnings to many meals. Please note that 8 of the grains listed below cook in 30 minutes or less. If you can have them cooking while putting a few other things together and herding the troops to set the table, pour drinks, etc., you can be ready with a fresh and healthy meal in about 30 minutes!

COOKING WHOLE GRAINS (adapted from The Whole Grains Council[14])

Use 1 cup of	With this much H20	After boiling simmer for…	To yield this much cooked grain
Amaranth	2 cups	20 – 25 minutes	3.5 cups
Barley, hulled	3 cups	45 – 60 minutes	3.5 cups
Buckwheat	2 cups	20 minutes	4 cups
Bulgur wheat	2 cups	10 – 12 minutes	3 cups
Cornmeal (polenta)	4cups	25- 30 minutes	2.5 cups
Coucous (whole wheat)	2 cups	10 minutes (heat off after boiling, cover)	3 cups
Kamut	4 cups	Soak overnight, then 45 – 60 minutes	3 cups
Millet (hulled)	2.5 cups	25 – 35 minutes	4 cups

Baby Steps to Better Health / Baby Step #3

Use 1 cup of	With this much H20	After boiling simmer for…	To yield this much cooked grain
Oats (steel cut)	4 cups	20 minutes	4 cups
Quinoa (keen-wah)	2 cups	12 – 15 minutes	3 cups
Rice (brown)	25 cups	25 – 45 minutes	3 – 4 cups
Rye berries	4 cups	Soak overnight then, 45 – 60 minutes	3 cups
Sorghum	4 ups	25 – 40 minutes	3 cups
Spelt berries	4 cups	Soak overnight, then 45 – 60 minutes	3 cups
Wheat berries	4 cups	Soak overnight, then 45 – 60 minutes	3 cups
Wild rice	3 cups	45 – 55 minutes	3.5 cups

CHAPTER 3B: Baby Step 3B - Stock a Healthy Pantry

INFORMATION: The food industry is not in business for your health.

Publicly owned companies that produce food are governed by the same principles that guide other publicly owned companies. They are supposed to make money for their stockholders. Profit, not your health and well-being, is the bottom line. Clearly these companies must be careful not to cause identifiable, outright harm or they will be sued. But, like the tobacco companies, they are not necessarily forthcoming with information about their products or ingredients, AND they often utilize their own research firms to find what they want found and shared with the public. I know I'm sounding pretty cynical, but it is true. So the more mystery involved in your food (i.e., where it came from, what those ingredients are, what they break down into, whether they were produced in a way that leaves nasty residuals behind), the more likely you are to be consuming something that is there to influence buying habits and not health, or is simply there to lower manufacturing costs, regardless of its impact on your health.

Large corporations are very good at what they do – which is sell stuff. There is an entire book about how the food industry has gone out of its way to discover the ingredients that will hook you on their products[15]. I do mean hook... as in addict. Therefore, the less processed food you eat, the better off you are. It is SO much easier to accomplish that intention when you don't have processed food readily available. It is easier to accomplish once you've discovered some time saving healthy recipes and tips that can increase the number of times per week that your family eats real food. It would be very difficult to remove all processed food from your diet overnight, but remember - the goal is to improve our healthy eating habits one baby step at a time so that the changes are less stressful and more likely to be permanent.

REFLECTION: on contents of pantries, refrigerators and freezers

This is a true reflection of the contents of our own pantries, refrigerators and freezers. Our voices are often mixed in this book, but in this case Little Sis is in italics and Bigg Sis is in normal type for the rest of the Reflection section.

In Baby Step 3, Bigg Sis (against all rationality) offered you all a look into our pantries. Mercy. Despite my many fine qualities, I have to admit to being somewhat (and I am being uncharacteristically generous with myself here) organizationally challenged. But since my sister showed you HERS, I guess I have to show you MINE. Yikes.....

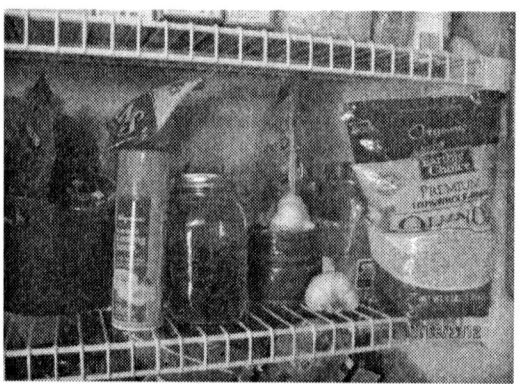

Now that I've given you a visual, let's talk about what's in that puppy. Bigg Sis was kind enough to compile her pantry list first (since she offered, it only seemed fair) so I will share hers and add the things that I keep in my pantry that she hasn't included. Before we get to the lists of ingredient staples that we both keep on hand in order to ensure that we can cook real food, we both have some processed bits to confess, just so's you know that the road just keeps going before all of us and neither of us would dream of claiming to be at the finish line.

Mr. Little Sis and I keep coffee and tea on hand as both parents in this house are nowhere near ready to drop that crutch. We keep a few boxes of cereal (all under 5g of sugar per serving or they must be mixed with a SUPER low sugar cereal). We also keep the occasional box of whole wheat and white cheddar macaroni and cheese for Daddy's traveling and Mommy's had enough emergencies. In addition we usually have a package of store bought cookies (of the fig newton variety) to bridge the gap between baking bursts. There are also our beloved Triscuits. :-)

Can't believe I didn't mention Triscuits! We also keep these simple gems on hand. You want to peep in my pantry as well, eh? I'm going to leave out the staples like coffee and tea (decaf for me because I'm a little *(Bigg Sis is also generous with herself)* high strung shall we say?), but I'd be remiss if I did not share a few smudges on an otherwise clean enough to put the scraps on record...I do keep a steady supply of boxed cereal in my pantry. I get brands with no additives / organic once in a while and all on sale – but there you have it. I do make granola and we do eat hot cereal but we all like a little bit of boxed cereal with fruit as a bedtime snack and it makes a great mix in for trail mix. But that's it... uh, well...except for the not-as-bad-for-you natural tortilla and potato chips that my son takes to school. There, confession complete! Oh wait –one more thing, (how many more things are there you wonder?)... I use tofu sometimes. Technically tofu is a processed food, because unfortunately it does not grow on trees. Now I'm done! I feel cleansed and refreshed, and I hope some of you are feeling better as well... We all have skeletons in the pantry, don't we? Here are the items that I always keep stocked so I'll be prepared to make healthy food rather than get fast food or eat something pre-made.

GRAINS:
oats - lots of great uses for these, including raw oats soaked overnight(p134)
brown Rice
quinoa -try Hearty, Hot and Healthy(p137) for breakfast
millet
whole grain pasta
bulgur

DRIED BEANS:
black beans, navy beans, pinto beans, garbanzos, etc.
lentils
mung beans for sprouting

Part of Bigg Sis' pantry is not IN the pantry. Pretty jars, eh?

Baby Steps to Better Health / Baby Step #3

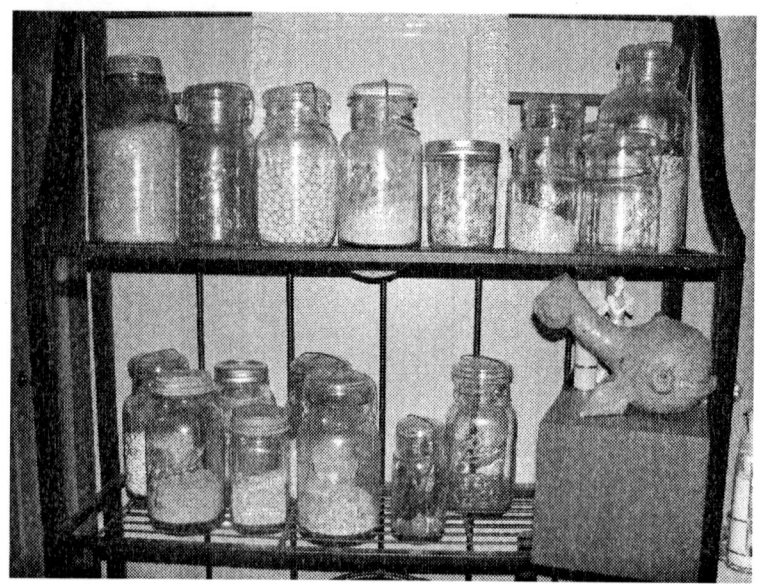

CANNED GOODS:
canned beans
canned (or boxed) tomatoes and paste
canned pineapple
artichoke hearts
olives

CONDIMENTS:
Bragg's Liquid Aminos (I use in place of soy sauce)
sesame oil
olive oil
safflower oil
salsa
mustard
broth/stock
ketchup – I buy organic with no added sugar
rice vinegar
balsamic vinegar
coconut oil

VEGGIES:
sweet potatoes
Yukon gold or red potatoes
onions
winter squash when it's cold out

Baby Steps to Better Health / Baby Step #3

NUTS & DRIED FRUIT:
Cashews
peanuts
sunflower seeds
almonds
pecans, pumpkin seeds
raisins
other dried fruit purchased on sale ;-) *cherries are a favorite of ours, dates, occasionally figs*

REFRIGERATOR:
Eggs
whole grain bread
milk (be it dairy, almond, soy or coconut!)
cheese (be it dairy or vegan)
carrots and celery
apples
whole wheat tortillas
flax meal for vegan eggs
sunflower cheese(p121)
hummus(p123)

FREEZER:
whole grain flour
frozen peas, green beans, corn, spinach
nuts (pecans, walnuts, almonds – all raw)
frozen herbs
frozen leftover pancakes

Whew. When you list it all it seems like a lot, but it's really NOT so much. And truthfully, neither of us ALWAYS has all of these things. I don't keep this list in my pocket and freak out when one item is low. This is simply the list of things that we have discovered make it easy for us to keep our promise to ourselves to NOT turn to takeout dinners out of desperation. It would be lovely to have oodles of time for every dinner, but that ain't life, and some nights there's a shortage of time AND patience. Being stocked up on REAL ingredients makes these nights a lot easier to face healthfully and economically. Hang in there and we'll show you how.

ACTION: Stock a Healthy Pantry

Pick 2 recipes that are fast and easy that your family enjoys and make sure that the items required to make those dinners are on a permanent shopping list. A permanent shopping list is a short list of items that you almost always buy when you go to the store. It might be a few cans of beans, a fresh veggie and fruit, milk, eggs…. Things that you can always fall back on and you would hate to get home and realize you forgot them. A permanent shopping list lives in the wallet of all of the shoppers in the house so they can whip it out when stopping for an item or two and perhaps pick up some of those items as well so you will all be ready for the next hurried meal…which will probably be any minute!

Baby Steps to Better Health / Baby Step #3   34.

Wrapping Up the Action: Baby Steps for Baby Step #3B

3B-1) Choose 1 or 2 recipes from recipes you already use that do not use processed food OR

3B-2) See a short list of easy and fast in the <u>expansion section</u>.

3B-3) Make a grocery list and distribute to shopping age family members.

3B-4) Choose when you will next make your real food meals.

(Available in Workbook)

EXPANSION:

First this section provides a short list of easy / fast recipes and then some more info on how we all got in this chemicalized, unhealthy pickle in the first place.

SHORT LIST OF EASY DINNERS:

All of these are available in the recipe section at the end of the book

Chickpea and Cashew Tikka Masala(p165)
Combo Bowl Sauce (for grains and veggies)(p207)
30 minute bean and bulgur chili(p162)
Sweet Potato / Apple / Oat Nuclear Incident(p140)
Chickpea Salad Sammies(p165)
Bellywarming American Black Bean Soup(p227)
Creamy Walnut Pesto(p202)
Spinach Chickpea Burgers(p193)
Lentil, Mushroom and Sweet Potato Soup(p232)
Cold Sesame Noodles(p168)
Garlic Mushrooms(p213)
Healthy Bechamel with Kale and Mushrooms(p172)
Nofredo Orzo with Chickpeas, Peas, and Kale(p181)

It's Not You, It's Them

The release of Michael Moss' book <u>*Salt Sugar Fat: How the Food Giants Hooked Us*</u> has prompted a flood of news stories. Moss is a New York Times reporter and a Pulitzer Prize winner. The guy has street cred as an investigator. I've not yet read the book; however, I've read the excerpt provided by Moss to the NYT Magazine. I also heard Moss interviewed on NPR's 'Fresh Air'. Moss' revelation confirms the worst of my concerns about the producers of processed and convenience foods. The long and short of it is that when you feel like you can't stop eating Oreos, that's because you very nearly can't. It's not you, it's them.

Moss reveals that in 1999 the Vice President of Kraft addressed CEOs of the other leading food producers and laid out his concerns about the growing obesity crisis and the increasingly clear links between highly processed foods and some of America's biggest health threats. This individual worried about his industry's culpability both from a moral and a financial perspective – we could get sued people. The response of his peers? We are responsible to our shareholders. We've spent a long time figuring out exactly how much salt, sugar and fat to use to ensure that consumers will buy our products and we cannot risk the loss of market share that would surely result from a change in practices. Let me say that part again: we are beholden to our shareholders. Guess who's not in that sentence? You (unless of course you are a majority shareholder in General Mills or something).

Let me be clear, I am aware that companies who make food are for-profit companies. I realize that this is the arena in which they are making their living. Somehow, however, the brazenness of the shareholder beholden-ness shocked me. The implications of the food industry's refusal to consider health crises in food formulation are vast. For me, the takeaway from Moss' revelations is two-fold: 1) processed and packaged food has been scientifically researched and developed to maximize taste, addiction, and profit, and 2) the onus of providing your body with nutritious food falls entirely on you.

Profit and Food Products

The research behind the formulation of most modern processed food was actually performed by scientists working for the military. Military rations must withstand unusual conditions (unpredictable temperature ranges, long term storage) and they must be nearly instant in preparation. The problem that the military discovered in the 70s was that the rations were so gross that military personnel were actually refusing to eat them. I don't think I need to tell you how problematic a lack of calories might be in a wartime situation. So the military sought out the help of science. How can we make food that tastes good enough to eat and that will still hold up to the conditions that wartime activities might impose? The answer was to add a whole mess of sugar, salt, and fat.

Researchers found the "bliss point" of sugar – the amount of sugar that actually makes you feel happy and that stimulates additional desire for food (ain't sugar grand?). Sugar can also improve the appearance of various foods. This all worked very well for military rations; and then the same research got applied to EVERYBODY's food. Food that doesn't need to withstand those crazy and unpredictable conditions, food for people who are not exerting themselves physically all day and who have other choices; food that people could eat everyday for their entire lifetime rather than temporarily in an emergency situation. The food industry has systematically added salt, sugar, and fat to food to find the magic amount which will encourage you to buy it, eat too much of it, feel like crap, and then buy it again. It's not you, it's them. They have taken advantage of you and your biological wiring to make more money.

Being a Nutrition Consumer

I get the feeling that most of us assume that the products that are available to us in stores are safe to eat. We have a Food and Drug Administration; there are rules and regulations about food production and sale. We see that there are recalls from time to time, so obviously somebody is ensuring that our food is good for us. This couldn't be further from the truth. Sure, there are rules and regulations and the occasional recall, but these are all about things like E. Coli, Listeria, and substances like melamine. They are not about diabetes and heart disease. Nobody has insisted that food producers actually make food that won't hurt you over the course of a lifetime. The healthy functioning of your body, the physical quality of your life is not their concern. The rate of your consumption is their concern. The number of packages of salt, sugar, and fat is what they are about.

When you make a large purchase for your family, say a car, you likely do a bit of research. You find out which cars have good safety records. You find out which cars don't break down. You find out which car is going to give you the maximum bang for your available buck. You do all of this because you KNOW that the car sales folks are NOT looking out for your best interest; they're trying to sell as many cars as they can. They're trying to increase their profit margin. They're trying to keep their shareholders happy. Does this sound familiar to you?

In the face of food choices, it's clear that there is only one answer to the problem. It's not them... it's you. It's us. It is up to us to find out which foods are safe for our families; it is up to us to find out which foods will provide our bodies with the fuel that they need to run efficiently and with maximum reward. It is up to us to find out which foods will give us the most bang for our nutritional buck. Just because it's cheap doesn't mean it will do what you want and need it too – we know this is true when we shop for other goods. We must assume it is true about our food. We must assume that food producers will do what they feel they must to get us to buy their food, and that the choices they make may not be the ones we would make if we were involved in that conversation. Food is a commodity. It is a good that is sold for profit. It is not, apparently, a public good.

What To Do?

It's clear that a desire to be healthy should lead us to learning about food products, reading labels, and preparing real, whole foods. I know there are challenges, but let's not lose sight of the fact that, in the paraphrased words of Michael Moss: maybe cooking real, whole food isn't as inconvenient as the food companies would have us think it is. Maybe the boxes that save us SO much time only save us ten minutes. Maybe we'd feel so much better cooking our own food that we wouldn't care that it took 10 minutes longer. Maybe over time our cooking skills would catch up with our schedules through practice and none of it would take longer than those boxes and frozen items that are scientifically engineered to be addictive. Maybe we've been sold more than convenience food, maybe we've been sold a bill of goods about how hard it is to make our own real food. What if we all decided to find out? What kind of food would they make next? I think it's time for a grand experiment. If you'd like to play along, give real food a try. The internet and your local library are chock full of resources for researching the most important purchases you make, the fuel for your body, the driver for your brain, the energy for your spirit. Caveat emptor. Let the buyer beware. Let the buyer be informed. Let the buyer eat food, real food.

CHAPTER 4: Baby Step 4 - Guiding Loved Ones on the Journey : Attitude is Everything

INFORMATION: *They won't eat that!*

There are good reasons why people don't adopt healthier eating habits, but they can all be overcome with information and less effort than you might think.

I can't tell you how many times I've heard it: "I want to eat healthier, but my kids (partner, whomever) won't eat that food." Everyone who said it was 100% certain that this was true. The only thing I am 100% certain about as regards feeding others healthy food is that if you don't have it/make it/serve it, they certainly won't eat it.

Changing our own eating habits is hard; convincing others that changing their eating habits is a fun group project can be daunting at best, but the difficulty of the task doesn't mean it isn't worth the effort. The Sis sisters have enlisted our families (immediate and in some cases extended) in our pantry transformations and we have some ideas that just might help you do the same. The truth is that, as with any meal, eating real food is easier and more enjoyable when you do it with the people that you love.

So here we approach the core of Baby Step 4: just as eating healthier foods requires you to be more conscious of what you're eating and how you're making it, so too, rallying the troops will require an evolution in consciousness about food. You must be the leader in the movement to develop an attitude of adventure, experimentation and gratitude surrounding food and mealtimes in your home.

REFLECTION: *A positive attitude greases the wheels of change.*

I can't speak for everybody, but when I embark on a new venture that I'm enthusiastic about, I want to share it. I want to share it with everybody and I (unreasonably) want everyone to be as excited as I am… It's sweet, isn't it? The cold water of reality is a bit uncomfortable. Just because I'm enthused doesn't mean they will be. My loved ones' priorities might be entirely different from mine and the mental steps I've taken to prepare myself for this wonderful new transformation have not necessarily been their mental steps. If we can agree that baby steps are an effective tool for making changes in our eating habits, we must remember that those we wish to encourage (and feed) deserve the same gracious and gentle introduction to foods with which they are unfamiliar and that these new foods may not initially inspire them. Does this mean don't try? No, no it doesn't. It may mean don't try ALL the time. It may mean be ready to see consumption without complaint (but no real enjoyment) as progress over grousing. It may mean lovingly saying that you understand when deep inside you'd like to remove all the plates from the table and tell everybody to…. okay, that's just me now and again – I know, it's not pretty, and I know it won't help. So we press on friends!

Baby Steps to Better Health / Baby Step #4

> *4a) Have the loved ones I'm trying to bring with me on this journey expressed an interest in following this path?*
>
> *4b) Do the loved ones I'm trying to encourage tend to be interested in change or trying new things?*
>
> *4c) Assuming everyone won't be as excited as I am or as open to new foods as I'd like, what baby steps am I willing to view as progress for them when it comes to improving our diet together?*
>
> *(Available in Workbook)*

ACTION: *Baby Step # 4 - Attitude is Everything*

Our suggestions for fostering a new food culture with loved ones fall into three basic categories:

1) The Use and Acceptance of Baby Steps as Progress,

2) Attitudinal Adjustments,

3) Education,

Category 1) The Use and Acceptance of Baby Steps as Progress

Progress towards what? That's what you must identify to help get them on board. Whether they would like to be healthier so they: don't get sick as often; lose weight; look healthier; perform better at sports; or just want to feel better and have more energy, identifying a reason to make a change will help them make a change. There is evidence (available in the expansion section at the end of this chapter) that children who eat healthful family meals eat more healthfully away from the family, do better in school, and have fewer drug and alcohol problems. You can explain this to everyone as well. You can also present your own reasons for wanting to eat more healthfully and ask them for help in meeting your own goals. Then explain the Baby Steps program. Most people would rather change things a bit at a time than change everything at once, so assure them that their favorite food is not necessarily on the chopping block.

Action #1: You must be the leader and perhaps the tyrant here. Give your family some reasons to want to be healthier and designate one meal per week to be healthier food night/ or healthier entree or side dish night if you need a gentler step.

Category 2) Attitudinal Adjustments

Family mealtime means different things to different people and for many folks time around the table is comfort. When we are trying new foods, it's not always so very comfortable. So rather than highlighting the comfort of familiar foods, we must highlight the adventure of trying new things. This can be particularly challenging with little people. I get it, really I do. But again, if we give up, all we can be sure of is that they will NEVER try the new food. If we persist and attempt to make it fun, who knows what will happen?

This is what we remind our sweeties of. If you don't TRY it, you'll never know. We then remind them of the foods they've tried and discovered how delicious they are. If we're trying a dish that highlights flavors from another culture, we talk about that place and the role that this food plays there. We take an adventure. When they are adventurous with their food, we lavish them with praise. Bigg Sis had a great idea that I think we will implement – the adventurous eater medallion. We may also try adventurous eating hats. Occasionally, in desperation, we appeal to their sibling rivalry and have a race to try the new food. I can't say the last method encourages delightful table manners, but it does seem to work for getting the new food in the mouth.

In addition to the positive role that adventurousness and competition can play, there is no way to overstate the importance of gratitude at the table. Mr. Little Sis has instituted a fabulous family tradition at the beginning of our meals. As head chef, I occasionally become discouraged by the cajoling that feeding twin 7 year olds can require. When we sit down to eat, Mr. Little Sis immediately says, "Thank You Mommy, for making such a wonderful meal for us." The twins usually follow on quickly, even if they are mid-complaint or moving stuff around to see what's under there and icky-face-making.

The most interesting thing about it is that once they've said thank you, they rarely return to the complaints, at least not with volume and vigor, which helps keep the mood at the table a little lighter, and prevents them from discouraging one another from trying new foods. Highlighting the importance of gratitude in a positive way, "We are so fortunate to have this healthy and nourishing food, and to be able to enjoy it together," over the "There are starving kids all over the world who would be happy to eat that _____," rightly changes the focus at the table from whether or not the meal meets every individual's expectations to mealtime as a time to come together and recharge.

Action #2: Establish adventurousness and gratitude by asking for it and acknowledging it. Reward adventurousness and model gratitude.

Category 3) Education

Different strategies work for different people. Some like the games (my daughter) and some need the rationale. I am still making this meal even though you've expressed it's not your favorite because it has ingredients in it that do _____ inside your body. Anything that helps my son's allergies will go in his mouth. Guaranteed. It is difficult NOT to take advantage of that knowledge. We've also talked a great deal about why I pack their lunches and why I don't include many of the things their friends eat regularly.

I marvel at the lack of pushback on this. The kids occasionally express their severe deprivation (along with a host of injustices that I have perpetrated), but they also, I've found, are able to make healthy choices that I am confident they would not make if we didn't share so much food information.

I've discovered that when they are offered a treat at a party, they limit themselves, without my saying anything. They tell me when they've had a surprise goody at school or with friends so that I can make adjustments to what I give them for the rest of the day. They GET IT. When they're older and they ask about McDonald's (or whatever) rather than toeing the line on that front as they do now, perhaps we'll sit down and watch "SuperSize Me" together. My husband and I watched several food documentaries before we embarked on the last round of dietary changes, discussed the information we found, researched the questions that remained. Just as I need information to make a big change, so too do the loved ones in my life.

Action #3: Educate your loved ones by telling them why you are doing what you are doing.

Wrapping up the Action: Baby Steps for Baby Step #4

So your Baby Step? What should you do? You should consider your cohorts and companions and try (gently and patiently) to get'em on board. Your life will be easier; your food will be healthier; and your table will be a place of adventure, experimentation, and gratitude while you tackle another pantry swap, or try a new recipe. Baby Steps for you, Baby Steps for them. It worked for all of us once, right?

4-1) Establish baby steps with your family by designating one meal per week to be healthier food night/ or healthier entree or side dish night if you need a gentler step.

4-2) Establish adventurousness and gratitude by asking for it and acknowledging it. Reward adventurousness and model gratitude.

4-3) Educate your loved ones by telling them why you are doing what you are doing.

(Available in workbook)

EXPANSION: *Family meals improve more than nutritional health.*

One of my favorite opportunities to roll my eyes is provided by scientific studies that have 'discovered' the obvious. For instance the article, "Why is it easier to see someone close than far away?" *Psychonomic Bulletin & Review*, Feb. 2005, did indeed prove that it is harder to see someone when they are farther away. So I was sure that it would be easy to find evidence that eating dinner together is a positive action for family health and interaction. What I didn't expect to find was the abundance of evidence showing many and various positive effects of family dinners on the lives and health of children and teenagers.

Studies indicate that an increase in the number of family dinners eaten together is correlated with an increase in academic success, improvement in individual nutritional choices, and healthier physical development[16]. As an advocate of healthy eating who has noticed the impact of good nutrition on the behavior of my own child (and on myself), I shouldn't be surprised. I just wasn't prepared for the definitive nature of the evidence. The findings, which show increases in many higher levels of nutrients in those who eat more family dinners, also showed that young people who eat more family dinners, and are therefore better nourished, make more healthful food choices when away from home. Hey! Maybe they do listen to us sometimes! I have been assuming that I will lose control over what my son eats as he gets older. Perhaps the groundwork has been laid for him to make at least SOME good choices and will be solidified through simply eating dinner together as often as possible.

Equally promising for parents' ability to positively impact their children's lives in our busy culture, was the finding of an inverse relationship between family dinners and the use of tobacco, alcohol and marijuana[17]. The same study that found this relationship, also found that more family dinners reduced the risk of depressive symptoms and suicide involvement after controlling for family connectedness[18]. In other words, in two families with an equal rating of connectedness, the family that eats together is less likely to have a depressed or suicidal teenager.

Okay, okay, so we know it's a good idea, but eating more family meals together is easier said than done. We have gotten used to a mad pace that includes driving from place to place and eating 'convenience foods.' Do not succumb to the notion that you cannot change your current behavior patterns! As Little Sis points out above, you do KNOW that if you don't provide healthier food, they certainly will not eat healthier food. And it might not surprise you, but it might encourage you to know that another scientific study, funded by the National Institute of Aging, found that older beagles fed a healthy diet and given plenty of exercise performed nearly as well as younger ones on cognitive tests[19]. In other words, you *can* teach an old dog new tricks (as long as they are well nourished and well rested). It really is not surprising that healthy diet was involved in sustaining cognitive ability – brains need nutrients too!

We will continue to explore ways to help you find the time, recipes and motivation to enjoy more healthy meals to your family as we progress through the Baby Steps. If you need a refresher, head on back to an earlier Baby Step. Ask someone in your family to read this book as well, or to research the effects of healthy food on our lives. As we've discussed, they are many and varied and all of them do a body, and a family, good.

CHAPTER 5: Baby Step #5 - A Plan for Feeling and Looking Better

INFORMATION: You are ready to make a plan!

You now have enough information to make a plan. A plan will help you think through how you'd like to change your eating habits and to set goals and a timeline for yourself, which will help you be more successful in making real changes.

This time you are providing the information. Perhaps you've had enough of listening to us anyway? And we suspect that you're getting a little weary of legwork. You've experimented with a swap, you've kept a food journal, you've investigated your pantry, and you've thought for a bit about how to get those with whom you eat on board with the idea of a new approach to food. You didn't realize you'd already done so much, did you? Didn't do it all? That's okay. Jump in here, go back to the beginning and start there – whatever. There is no timeline.

The only due date I'd like to suggest is today. Do something today. No, don't wait until next week or next month... Waiting until next week or next month means losing a week or a month of taking baby steps down the road. There's no reason you can't get a little ahead of the game knowing that in addition to anything you're doing for others, you're also taking care of yourself. Convinced? Yay! It's time to make a plan....

REFLECTION: Don't Diet. Eat Food. Real Food.

When we decide to go on a diet, we are committing to a temporary state of restriction, usually in an attempt to achieve some sort of numerical change – a smaller waistline, a lower reading on the scale, a smaller clothing size. When we commit to a temporary state of restriction, we are admitting to the foregone conclusion that the results of that restriction – the number drop – will also be a temporary phenomenon.

> *5a) Have you ever gone on a restrictive diet before?*
>
> *5b) How did it go?*
>
> *5c) Did you get results?*
>
> *5d) Did the results last?*
>
> *5e) Did you consider it a success?*

Baby Steps to Better Health / Baby Step #5

(Available in Workbook)

You cannot return to the way you normally eat and maintain those lower numbers. It doesn't work. If in the past you've made a weight loss resolution, or a healthy eating resolution that was based on limiting your intake, you already know this is true. Simply restricting what you eat also doesn't guarantee that the food that you DO eat will actually nourish you.

When we decide to change the way that we eat, we are committing to a higher level of consciousness about what we eat in an attempt to eat food that is more healthful and that provides our bodies with more of what they require. We have found that a body that is getting what it needs is far less likely to torment us with the cravings that often drive us to eat unhealthy foods. When we decide to change the way we eat, we are committing to caring for our bodies and our health, and are therefore also committing to caring for those around us who love us and cherish us. When we decide to change the way that we eat, we open ourselves to the joy of living healthfully and the adventure of eating new and abundant real foods.

> *5f) Do you have specific concerns about your health or your family's health?*
>
> *5g) What are they?*
>
> *5h) List 5 healthy foods that you like.*
>
> *(Available in Workbook)*

If you're ready, we'll help you take those steps that will get you eating and feeling great in a way that works for you, with changes that YOU choose according to your timeframe. This is YOUR plan; it's YOUR body. You should be the one to decide what to put in it, thoughtfully and consciously, using ingredients that aren't invented in a lab. And you will find that the food you put in that body can be both succulent and healthful, both sublime and invigorating, both yummy and nourishing. Because real food is delish and it does your body good. Don't diet; Eat Food, Real Food.

ACTION: Planning Baby Steps to Look and Feel Better

Gather your stuff. Get that food journal. Open that pantry door. Peek in the refrigerator. Your mission is to make a list of foods that you'd like to baby step right out of your diet. No, you don't need to come up with a specific number. And yes, we will help you figure out which ones to start with if you're not sure. Let's see if we can't make some progress with a few simple questions/suggestions for places to start.

Baby Steps to Better Health / Baby Step #5

1) As you look at your food journal, is there something that you know is unhealthy and that you eat regularly for the sake of convenience or to treat yourself? Perhaps you have a soda habit or a frappuccino addiction. These are perfect places to start – a food that is not a meal, it's offering no nutrition, and it's loaded with sugar. Am I telling you to ditch them altogether forever? No. Do the best you can. Cut them out, cut them down, wean yourself, swap them out for something healthier. Whatever a baby step is to you... do that.

> *5i) Fess up. What is that something you know is unhealthy but you eat regularly?*
>
> *5j) How can you cut back?*
>
> *5k) When will you start?*
>
> *(Available in Workbook)*

2) As you consider your food choices, does carry out or fast food play a major role in your lunch or dinner meal planning? Set a goal for eating one more home cooked meal or one more brown bagged lunch per week than whatever your current total is.

> *5l) Does Fast Food figure into lunch or dinner regularly?*
>
> *5m) Decide to eat one or more home cooked meals per week than what you currently do. How many will it be? It's okay to start with 1!*
>
> *5n) Which meal(s) will you substitute real food for?*
>
> *(Available in Workbook)*

3) As you examine that pantry you've already peeped in, take notice of the number of packaged snacks. This is an excellent place to experiment with some snack swaps or learning to make a homemade snack.

> *5o) Does your family rely on packaged snacks?*
>
> *5p) Will they eat nuts and dried fruit or apples?*
>
> *5q) Would you like to try baking once in a while?*

Baby Steps to Better Health / Baby Step #5   46.

(Available in Workbook)

4) As you peek in the fridge, take notice of the beverages that are available. How many of them are sweet? How many of them are juice or juice-like? Juice and juice-like drinks are another excellent place to get started. Remember, you don't have to throw it out (unless you want to, and I'm certainly not going to stop you). Cut the amount, cut the frequency, mix it with water, swap it for something healthier.

> *5r) How many sweetened beverages does each family member drink daily?*
>
> *5s) Do you need to find alternatives or will they drink water?*
>
> *5t) Who will have the hardest time with this change?*

(Available in Workbook)

Still not sure where to get started? Some basic categories you should consider: foods with a lot of sugar or corn syrup, foods that contain excessive fat (especially hydrogenated fats), foods that contain excessive sodium (in all its forms), and highly processed foods (like those that stay good for a REALLY long time), fast food. (There is more information about sugar, including a list of many of its pseudonyms, and why it is so bad in the expansion section at the end of this chapter.)

Overwhelmed? Don't be. You are going to make a plan, which is a great way to be normally whelmed ;-). Now is when you take all those answers and thinking and make a list of foods or food categories that you want to eliminate from your diet and plan when to do it. You don't have to do them all at once but acknowledging that you intend to eliminate them and that there is a larger picture may help you stick with the changes you are making

Once you've got a list of things you'd like to cut/limit/wean yourself off of, choose a starting place. Pick one of them and consider how you want to proceed. Limit the quantity? Swap it out? Cut it altogether? Your answer will be different from my answer – what is a baby step to you may seem like a huge leap to me. This is YOUR plan, not a test of your character, but a series of decisions you get to make for yourself.

Finally, write down the steps you're going to follow to get started on that change. If you're going to limit your quantity, write down how that's going to work – what's the new limit and what are you going to do to replace that item? If you're cutting a sweet treat in the middle of your work day, what are you going to either eat, or do, to replace that ritual? Write it down. Write down your start date (today) and then give yourself a goal date for reaching whatever your desired change is on that item. If you want to ditch chewy granola bars, write down when you're going to start (today), write down what you're going to do instead (there could be a few steps here), and write down the date by which you hope to be done changing this food habit. Does that mean you'll never eat one again? Maybe, but probably not. And if you choose to have one it's not the end of the world, or a total failure. It's a decision and you will have lots more opportunities to make decisions.

Wrapping Up the Action: Baby Steps for Feeling and Looking Better

5-1) Make a list of foods or food categories that you want to eliminate from your diet

5-2) Plan when to do it

5-3) Choose a starting place for the first one(s) on your list

5-4) Write down the steps for elimination or reduction

> **(Available in Workbook)**

Remember, the key to healthy eating is making healthful decisions as often as you can. Establish a new pattern so that the chewy granola bar (or soda, or candy or drive through) is an exception rather than the rule. Open the door to improved nutrition and prepare to be wowed as your taste buds and your energy levels come back to life and you discover new satisfaction in eating for your health. And just in case you're wondering, this isn't all about what we cut out... we have plenty of suggestions about what to cut in. A little delish, morning, noon, and night comin' up.

INSPIRATION:

Sometimes it is inspiring to know that you are not on the journey alone. This is a list Little Sis shared right before the holidays – a notorious time to completely abandon all sensibility when it comes to food, right? This is one person's list. Yours will also be unique. Mine would not include caffeine because I am a naturally caffeinated person. It would however include sweets and other things as well! Most everyone's includes sweets I'm thinking! At any rate – here is an insight into part of Little Sis' journey.

Little Sis said her current list looks like this:
caffeine (UGH)
salt on the plate
afternoon sweet

So am I going to do all of these at once? Maybe, but I won't cut them all out. For my caffeine problem, I'm switching from two large mugs of my beloved coffee to one of coffee and one of black tea. The next step will be to switch the black tea out for green tea. Then black tea in the a.m., green tea in the afternoon… you get the picture. I have reduced caffeine before and in addition to the headache, I've found that being abrupt on this one makes me miserable and inflicts some level of misery on those around me… so I'm going to step it down, achieve my goal at a pace that allows me to make adjustments, allows me to tame my body's addiction over time without being a horrible grouch for the holidays.

I can tell you Little Sis is also a master of creating baked goods that are still very tasty but much lower in sugar and nasty fat & chemicals. This is a great way to fight the craving for sweets. Make them healthier sweets! Here is a list of some of the healthier sweets you'll find in our Desserts & Sweets section of the recipes(p143). Pumpkin Brownies (gluten free - GF); Celebration Krispies (GF); Healthy Pumpkin Cookies (GF); Walnut Crust Apple Pie (GF and easier than traditional!); Crancherry, Almond & White Chocolate Cookies; Sweet Potato Cookies with Walnuts and Dark Chocolate Chips; Intensely Good Banana Bread; Almond Lemon Jots (GF); Spicy Sweeties; and more!

If you need help with some swaps, go back and re-read Chapter 2: Baby Step 1. If you skipped the expansion section of that chapter maybe you need some cold hard facts to help you choose what to swap. You don't have to figure this all out yourself… and if you don't like your plan a week from now, know what you get to do? Change it. It's YOUR plan.

EXPANSION: Info about Sugar, Salt & Fat
Sugar – what could be wrong with Little ol' Sugah?

You're not going to like this any better than I do, but the first dangerous, and perhaps most abundant additive in processed food can be easily added right from the safety of your own kitchen teaspoon. Sugar. Sugar, also known as:

Agave nectar
Brown sugar
Cane crystals
Cane sugar
Corn sweetener
Corn syrup
Crystalline fructose
Dextrose
Evaporated cane juice
Fructose
Fruit juice concentrate

Glucose
High-fructose corn syrup
Honey
Invert sugar
Lactose
Maltose
Malt syrup
Molasses
Raw sugar
Sucrose
Syrup

Why so many names? There is the possibility that all of these various types of sugar have specific uses and hold up better under some preparation circumstances, temperatures, transport than do others. It is also true that ingredient lists begin with the most abundant ingredient and proceed in order to the least abundant ingredient. A food company that knew some of us would reject a product such as a breakfast cereal or granola bar or yogurt or cracker that had sugar as the first or second ingredient might appreciate the ability to divide sugar's presence among several or even many ingredients. Using different names for $C_{12}H_{22}O_{11}$ - that's sugar (sucrose) in chemistry language - would allow you to hide some of the sugar, both in language like malt syrup, and in amount. Not that anyone is doing that on purpose....

A couple of tips for detecting sugar: while checking labels on food, make sure that you look for words that end in 'ose' (this means sugar) and that you pay attention to the number of grams of sugar per serving (and what that serving size is) rather than only avoiding foods that have a sugar in the first or second place on the ingredient list. There are 4.5 grams of sugar in a teaspoon. You might find it easier to imagine the amount of sugar in a serving of processed foods if you convert the amount of sugar listed per serving into teaspoons.

Sugar has been denounced as the leading contributor to diabetes, heart disease and cancer in obese AND normal weight people. It isn't just 'health whacks' like us (that's what Bigg Sis' son calls us, God love him and his sweet tooth) making such claims. These pronouncements are coming from researchers at universities as well as organizations like the American Heart Association, the World Health Organization and the United Nations. Robert Lustig, a pediatric endocrinologist at the University of California in San Francisco, has stated that sugar should be regulated because it is just as dangerous as alcohol and tobacco and overly available to children.[20]

By now I'm sure you're wondering why I've included sugar as an additive. Isn't sugar natural? Sugar is not a natural food when it is removed from fruit (which used to be available to humans only part of the year), concentrated from plants such as sugar cane, sugar beets and maple trees, and used in excess. The human body has never seen such

Baby Steps to Better Health / Baby Step #5

an abundance of sugar and the increase in obesity and metabolic syndrome around the globe is linked to an increase in the intake of sugar-sweetened beverages (soda, vitamin water, sports drinks, energy drinks).[21] Sugar tastes good. Manufacturers want you to buy their processed foods. Without being able to offer freshness, food processors must grab you some other way and they do so by adding sugar to almost everything. And I do mean almost everything. Let's take a look at some surprising sources of sugar in processed food.

Ten Surprisingly Sugary Foods:[22]

1) breakfast bars : Nutri-grain bars contain 13 grams or almost teaspoons of sugar

2) vitamin water: 20 oz of Glaceau or Snapple anti-oxidant has 30 grams of sugar (about 7.5 tsp)

3) breakfast cereal

4) Prepared pasta sauce: Prego Marinara has 7 grams (almost 2 tsp) in ½ cup

5) bran muffin (20g in Starbuck's version)

6) dried fruit: varies by fruit and drying process, although we would argue that dried fruit in moderation is WAY better than candy

7) juice: varies widely, read the labels on your juice cocktails and juice blends

8) flavored yogurt: 6 ounces Yoplait strawberry has 27 grams (6 teaspoons) – ounce for ounce most flavored yogurts have as much sugar as a candy bar

9) instant oatmeal: 1 packet can contain up to 14 grams (over 3 teaspoons) of sugar

10) bottled iced tea: 22 ounces of Snapple Lemon Iced Tea has 36 grams of sugar (about 9 teaspoons).

Watch your condiments as well with Kraft Spicy Honey BBQ sauce – 2 Tbsp serving = 13 grams (about 3 tsp sugar) and Kraft 1,000 Island weighing in with 5 grams (a bit more than a teaspoon) in a 2 tablespoon serving.[23]

You must become an aisle-blocking, cart stopping, label reader in order to really understand the prevalence of sugar in processed foods. Go ahead and block the aisles. Make people wonder what is so fascinating on that label!

Unfortunately, artificial sweeteners are not a healthful answer. Artificial sweeteners may sound like a great idea, but "they don't lessen cravings for sugar and haven't demonstrated a positive effect on our obesity epidemic[24]," says Grotto, author of *101*

Foods That Could Save Your Life. And of course artificial sweeteners just don't fit the bill for real food, because they are not.

Fat – Jack Sprat didn't eat processed food.

The kind and amount of fat is where it's at. And although it can be complicated when you start researching, it is as simple as the rest of eating real food. Where did the oil come from? Oils from animals fed nasty, un-natural diets could be tainted with nasty, un-natural diet stuff!

According to many MDs and nutritional scientists like Neal Barnard, MD., T. Colin Campbell and Dr. Andrew Weil, animal fats and plant fats used in processed foods (trans fats or saturated fats) are fattening and inflammatory (cause inflammation and disease). When oils are processed they can lose nutritional value and acquire odd molecular forms and by-products that are bad for you. The Mayo Clinic website recommends choosing plant based oils based on their smoke point[25]. The smoke point is the temperature at which an oil begins to smoke and therefore break down and burn. Some of the by-products of smoking / burning oil are carcinogenic.

Type of Oil	High Smoke Point	Moderate smoke point	Low smoke point
Examples	Peanut, sunflower, safflower, sesame, corn, soybean, clarified butter, coconut oil (refined), avocado oil	Olive, canola, grapeseed, coconut oil (extra-virgin)	Flax seed, walnut
Uses	Frying, stir-frying	Sautéing over low to medium-high heat	Dressings and dips

The Sis sisters add to the consideration of smoke point of plant oils the same consideration we give to all foods. Where did it come from? Did it get doused with nasty chemicals in the process? Is it made from GMOs? Now this may or may not be a Baby Step for you down the road, but personally, we have been using coconut oil and avocado oil whenever possible – in place of butter in many recipes and for roasting and medium sautéing. Keep in mind of course that oils are dense in calories and should be kept to a minimum.

And finally, I found a Baby Step for the Sis sisters. Dr. Su Fairchild at the University of Kansas Medical Center website presents a great explanation of which oils suffer breakdown into unhealthy components[26]. Coconut oil is prominent in his list of healthy oils and is in vogue right now, but it is interesting to understand why and to realize the importance of how you store and use oils. Not everyone agrees with the notion that coconut oil is healthy because it is in fact a saturated fat.

Dr. Fairchild explains that polyunsaturated fatty acids (PUFA's) are "easily oxidized by oxygen and heat, and form much higher amounts of toxic lipid peroxides than saturated or monounsaturated oils. Exposure to high heat and oxygen during manufacturing, shipping and handling of these oils can be a factor in their quality even if you keep them closed up and at low temps at home. Dr. Fairchild suggests only cooking with oils that are less than 20% PUFA's and that are virgin and organic. Unfortunately this list consists of very few commonly used oils and organic oils are more expensive. Again, we offer information, not shaming. Remember to take Baby Steps and if you want more information, here is the list of oils that are less than 20% polyunsaturated fatty acids:

Pistachio oil (19% PUFA)
Cashew oil (17% PUFA)
Almond oil (17% PUFA)
Duck fat (13% PUFA, 1% cholesterol)
Lard (12% PUFA, 1% cholesterol)
Filbert oil (10-16% PUFA)
Avocado oil (10% PUFA)
Macadamia oil (10% PUFA)
Goose fat (10% PUFA, 1% cholesterol)
Palm oil (8% PUFA)
Olive oil (8% PUFA)
Butter (4% PUFA)
Ghee (4% PUFA, 2% cholesterol)
Cocoa Butter (3% PUFA)
Coconut oil (2-3% PUFA, 0% cholesterol)
Palm kernel oil (2% PUFA)

Some of these oils are not easy to come by but in our respective states of Maryland and Tennessee we both can purchase organic coconut oil and avocado oil.

Using other oils that are kept away from light, oxygen and heat in dressings or drizzling over food is okay. "Good fats and oils are very important, as they are required for absorption of fat soluble vitamins. The cells in our body also require good fats in the cell membrane. We cannot live without fat."[27]

Salt: You are the salt of the earth!

I have a salt problem. It's a hereditary problem. The Sis Sisters learned to pick up the salt shaker without tasting and cover first with multiple shakes of the salt in one direction, followed by multiple shakes of the salt at a 90 degree angle from our Dad.

Baby Steps to Better Health / Baby Step #5

Luckily for us, we are also blessed with low blood pressure, but who knows when that could change? Salt is linked to high blood pressure which is linked to cardiovascular disease[28]. Along with avoiding processed foods, you can try out new spices and new recipes that will expand your taste buds to recognize that the world offers more than salt as a wonderful savory flavor.

Salt hides on labels in the same ways sugar hides.... Spread out the salt content by name and you don't have to have salt as early in the label, thereby implying a lower salt content. Here are some other names for salt provided by KFL&A Public Health[29] (2007):
Monosodium glutamate (MSG)
garlic salt
onion salt
seasoning salt
kelp
sea salt
baking soda
baking powder
sodium chloride, or any chemical compound with sodium.

Even if you are a salt shaker, home-cooked foods are likely to be lower in salt than processed foods, so taking the real food route will help reduce your salt intake as well.

CHAPTER 6: Baby Step #6 - Develop New Food Habits and Rewards

INFORMATION - Behavior and habit are linked.
You can choose which habits you develop!

I heard a radio interview recently in which the interviewee had some really interesting, specific, and helpful things to say about habits. I immediately thought of changing the way we eat in terms of habits. So much of how we feed ourselves is habit driven, routine,, doing what we've always done. Habits can be hard to break. The Sis Sisters want to help and so does Jeremy Dean. He gives 10 tips for habit change that he covers in greater length in his new book *Making Habits, Breaking Habits*. I was delighted to see how many of his tips sounded like the kinds of things we suggest in our Baby Steps to Better Health series.

Dean's very first suggestion is "For Big Results, Think Small." He discusses the importance of making change in small, incremental, manageable and achievable bits. Sound familiar? Other themes that we both stress are repetition, tweaking (the same plan won't work for everyone), and replacing an undesirable behavior with one that is desirable rather than just trying to suppress the "bad" one. Yay! These are just a few of his tips – there are a total of 10 in his book. If you're trying to make some healthy changes, this guy just might have some insight for you. And there's nothing like having your advice validated by an official smart guy. ;-)

When it comes specifically to food and bad habits, we must consider our cultural habit of using food as a reward. When we perform well we celebrate with food. We 'deserve' a treat at the end of a hard day, don't we? We 'earned' a chocolate milkshake by cleaning out the garage. The only problem is that many of our celebratory foods are really not good for us. What kind of reward is that? Rewards aren't supposed to hurt, are they?

> *6a) What are some foods that you use as a reward?*
>
> *6b) What foods do friends and other family members use as a reward?*
>
> *6c) Do you use any non-food rewards in your home?*
>
> *(Available in Workbook)*

Baby Steps to Better Health / Baby Step #6

REFLECTION: *Pay attention to experiences of wellness and satisfaction*

The Sis sisters initially wrote this Baby Step at the end of December. January 1st is a popular but difficult time to make a change regarding food. I mean, on January 1st how many of us still have Christmas cookies in the house? Fudge? Candy canes? Chocolate? No wait. I always have chocolate in my house. In my defense it is dark chocolate and I limit myself to a small piece (2-3 squares from a bar) per day. What? How can you stop eating chocolate you ask? I'll answer that in a second, but would just like to point out that although the holidays bring all sorts of unusual treats into our homes, most of us always have a lot of 'food' on hand that is not healthy food. Some of it is for other people in the family, some of it is for a special occasion, some of it was on sale, some of it is just my favorite so quit bugging me, would ya?!

Food is a habit that is hard to break. No wait, that sounds ridiculous…. Poor food CHOICES can be a hard habit to break. Habits are hard to break. Food is a necessity and a wonderful part of life. We say it is time to develop new healthy food habits. They can be hard to break as well!

New healthy habits is the segue back to the chocolate. Yes there are Baby Steps regarding chocolate that you can feel good about. I certainly feel good about chocolate! I used to adore Reese's peanut butter cups and all manner of sugar-filled treats and candy. Switching to dark chocolate took time. I had to start with some in-between chocolate… kind of dark, kind of milk/wishy-washy Charlie Brown kind of chocolate. But as I developed new habits for snacks that were lower in sugar I began to find the more sugary versions WAY too sweet. In fact, when I eat a high sugar treat now, I feel really bad in about 10 minutes. No kidding. It's a great motivator to stay away from the crap, but it took some time to develop that sensitivity.

So my answer about having chocolate in the house without eating it is this. The less sugar in the chocolate, the more deeply satisfying is eating a reasonable amount, AND the less sugar, the less likely to cause craving for more. Reducing the amount of sugar you eat helps you recognize other delightful flavors: like the chocolate itself, like cinnamon, like lemon, like fruit! That is my experience. And it is experience that has guided us on our quest to eat more healthfully, and to achieve a degree of success towards that proposition. I got used to dark chocolate. I paid attention to it. I pay attention to how I feel after eating healthier food. Pay attention to what makes you feel badly, but also pay attention to experiences of wellness and satisfaction because they can help you change. Honor the good experiences and repeat them. Repeated experience develops habits. Paying attention to experience helps us develop healthy habits. Once you've paid attention and developed the new habit you just might find yourself choosing that piece of fruit over a piece of cake just because you've gotten used to doing it every day. It is simply what you do. You too can develop new habits and new rewards.

ACTION: Develop New Habits and Rewards

6d) Is there a hiding place for grown up food rewards?

6e) Do you ever enjoy your food reward with the TV off?

(Available in Workbook)

1) Make yourself a list of non-food rewards. One of mine is to step outside (when possible) smell the air and look for some birds or other wildlife. That always makes me feel better. A little break, no harmful intake. Then if I am really hungry, I can eat something that will nourish me in all my bird-loving glory.

Seriously, make a list. Little things, little treats… treats you can pay attention to like a cup of flavorful herb tea, a game of cards with your sweetie or friend, a flower or two to put in a vase where you'll see it, a bath with scented water, a few guilt free minutes reading a magazine, a quick call to a friend. Make a list because options are good and options can help you overcome old, harmful habits, but only when you think of and choose them.

If you're not ready to replace your sweet treats with activities, a smaller Baby Step is to reduce the amount of the unhealthy food you are using as a reward. One way of doing this is to enjoy this treat without distraction. Do NOT eat your bowl of ice cream or your dark chocolate in front of the TV set. When we eat in front of the TV, we do not appreciate our treat as much and before we know it, our beloved treat is gone and we don't even remember eating it which is not much of a reward, so, surely we deserve another shot at appreciating the reward we deserve so much. So we have some more. Yikes! Not a reward - a habit. Sit down with that smaller bowl of ice cream / piece of chocolate, whatever YOUR food reward is and look at it. Touch it. Smell it. Savor every slow bite. You will enjoy it more, it will take longer to eat and you will find the experience much more satisfying. Whatever the reward you choose from your list, food or non-food – savor it. It is a reward after all!

2) Place a copy of your reward list in several places – like the place(s) where you currently stash the sweet goods. Read it when you are tempted to indulge in an old habit. Another benefit to the list of non-food rewards is that when the habit rears its head, if you go get the list, or read your list, you have a chance to move beyond the initial impulse. Habits are in a way trained impulses. Given a little bit of time to think about the consequences of our habitual actions, we might make a better, or less bad, choice.

Baby Steps to Better Health / Baby Step #6

3) Close your eyes when you're sure that you 'deserve' that bag of Doritos or Reese's peanut butter cup, breathe, and count to 10. Then look around you wherever you are and decide what you are going to do next. Maybe the treat won't seem so important anymore, or you will acknowledge a healthier choice and 'treat' yourself well. You might even find that it helps to touch a few things and think about them and how grateful you are to have them. Realizing some blessings sometimes makes it easier to make healthy reward choices because you can see some of the rewards that already exist in your life.

Wrapping up the Action: Baby Steps for Baby Step #6

6-1) Make a list of non-food or smaller healthier food rewards.

6-2) Keep your list in several places where you can read it when you need an alternative.

6-3) Close your eyes, breathe and count to 10 before indulging your old unhealthy habit.

(Available in Workbook)

INSPIRATION: Investigating Habit Change

Sometimes I get super HONGRY and want to eat all the time. Habits I've developed can really play a big role in food choice on HONGRY days. I had a run of HONGRY days after the holidays recently and the habitual holiday cookie pass and grab became more of a face stuffing activity. As I recognized this (and began to feel the limits of my pants), I decreased my cookie intake. It was really difficult to cut back, and I couldn't figure out why I was feeling SO deprived for just passing up on a cookie or twelve. So very, very HONGRY. And then it struck me, the sweets weren't the only holiday slippage.

When I apply myself to a new initiative, I really go for it. Not much for half measures, this girl. Of course not much for finishing either but that's a different and way too long to finish – HA- story. When I made some pretty hefty dietary changes last spring, I really went for it. Eliminated a bunch of things systematically that I thought were making me feel blechy and upped the produce content of every plate and snack by A LOT. The new project enthusiasm made these big changes easy. I didn't feel deprived. I felt great and I did NOT feel HONGRY. So in examining my habits since the holidays I noticed that I was not only eating more sweets but I was eating less of the things I was snacking on before – veggies and fruit – produce. So I decided to run a little experiment.

For the past few days every time I got HONGRY I've grabbed some plant matter (mostly carrots because I really like them and they require so little fuss) and jammed it in my gaping gullet, a little pre-emptive produce (PEP) as Bigg Sis calls it. I haven't dictated to myself that there will be no more cookies, but I've instituted the same policy I have for my kids – if I'm hungry I should eat something REALLY nutritious first. Guess what? The HONGRY has calmed down to just hungry and the cookies are getting easier to pass up as my sweet tooth settles down again. Such a simple lesson that I learned a while ago, and yet in all the crazy holiday-ness I forgot one of the most important principles: your body needs food. If you only give it crap, you will be HONGRY.

How's it going for you? Finding yourself feeling deprived or HONGRY? What's going on the plate as you take your targeted indulgences off? Feed that body; feed it good. And when you've done a good thing, and are feeling really proud of yourself – go outside and look at the birds. Rewards are all around us – not just in the cookie tin.

EXPANSION

If you are someone who is inspired or motivated by books then we encourage you to look for a highly recommended or rated book on breaking habits. If that doesn't help you so much, it may help just to consider the extent to which habit is involved in your food intake. Understanding that you are fighting a habit and impulse and not just taste preference may make it easier to stick with your changes, even after a failure, or 2, or 5 ;-). Also consider how your taste preferences change over time. They can change. You can change. You can even eat healthy food and enjoy it.

CHAPTER 7: Baby Step 7 – How Convenient Are Convenience Foods?

INFORMATION – It isn't convenient just because 'They' say it is.

Elephant skin is so tough they call it 'hide'. Have you ever wanted your hands to be as soft as 'hide'? Ever heard admiration expressed as, "Oooh. This is as soft as an elephant's hide!" I'm guessing you haven't. Well, we at the pantry have been pushed up against the side of the elephant in our Baby Steps kitchen for a while and it's time for a breather. The bumpy, rough-hided elephant of which I speak, is TIME. While Einstein may not be bothered by the obstructive elephant of time because he understands the elephant much better than we do, there are only so many minutes in each day and trying to fit everything in can feel like an impossible task.

Maybe you're thinking, "Finally, you are going to talk about time….It's about time because I haven't got much, and I'm thinkin' all this cooking you do takes a lot of TIME!" I hear your shouts of frustration rending the space-time continuum…. Okay, maybe it's not that bad and we do not need to pull in some disciple of Einstein to address that, but we acknowledge that many people feel that they don't have time to cook healthy food. We want to address the reality of your limited time in Baby Step 7: ReCon Convenience. For this step, we are all about figuring out time as it relates to eating healthfully. Many people assume that cooking and eating real food takes a long time and that buying carry-out and convenience food allows a busy person to get dinner on the table faster. We want to challenge these assumptions, and help you figure out your own time as it relates to how you eat. We are willing to bet that it doesn't take as long as you think it does to eat healthfully!

REFLECTION:

A few questions to ask yourself:

> *7a) Where is my time currently wasted in regards to food procurement and preparation?*
>
> *7b) Where is my time wasted when I think I'm actually saving time?*
>
> *7c) Where will I find the time difference between pulling something out of the freezer to heat up and preparing something with real food ingredients from scratch.*

(Available in Workbook)

And finally, will the Sis sisters come clean my house for me on a weekly, or I'd even settle for bi-weekly, basis?

I'll take care of that last one. No.

Okay that was a bit harsh. We might clean yours if you'd clean ours, as it might at least be more interesting to clean someone else's house for a change. But let's get back to Baby Step 7. We've given questions 7a-7c a longer think and want to share some of our thinks with you... Our answers to these questions constitute your action plan for this Baby Step. We know that limited time is a real elephant of a problem so there's a lot of explanation here, and quite a few steps – but they are steps. Take them one at a time, preferably more forward than back. The action steps will be listed again at the end of the section.

ACTION: How Convenient Are Convenience Foods?

Question #1) Where is my time currently wasted in regards to food procurement and preparation?

We've identified some of our time wasters and I bet you've whiled away several days of your life in much the same manner!

Time Waster A) Too many trips to the grocery store. (This was a biggie for us).

POSSIBLE SOLUTION: Extend the period of time between grocery store trips. Plan your meals for a period of nights, make a shopping list and get what you need in fewer trips. We currently aim for 2 trips to the store a week. One main trip after planning and another trip later in the week for the produce that won't make it a week and/or the things I forgot! Better than the previous 3 – 4 times per week.

STEP: come up with a plan for planning.

Decide when you will make meal plans.
Then decide where you will keep the plan, if and how you will share your meal plan and the grocery list that goes with it. If you have children you can likely see the advantage of sharing the plan (so you don't have to answer THE QUESTION 300 times a day) or keeping it a secret (so you don't have to hear the editorial comments that will surely follow). Shared plans and grocery lists, however, can be very useful in getting real helpful help if you are looking to dole out some food responsibilities. We'll discuss this more in a later step. At the end of the chapter we'll also share how we use meal plans to cut time in food preparation..

Baby Steps to Better Health / Baby Step #7

Time Waster B) Not planning for or making use of leftovers:

Always, always, always make extra food and especially extra grain (rice, barley, quinoa, etc.) as these can be used in future meals (including some really fast and healthy breakfasts). Leftovers rule! What is faster – making a sandwich for a lunchbox or placing leftovers in a container? This can be done while cleaning up the evening meal as well…. Pack some leftovers for Mom, some for Dad and some for whichever kid will eat that particular leftover in their lunch.

STEP: Make sure you have containers for holding leftover meals and grains.

Plan a meal in which you will make extra and use the leftovers in containers for lunches or for another meal in a few days. If you write your meal plan to include 2 meals that use the same grain you can make enough for both at one time and store the extra grain.

Time Waster C) Going it alone – (I am woman, hear me roar and/or 'nobody else does it right!')

Invite help. It's not just what we eat that can be governed by habit but how food gets purchased and prepared. If you've always been the one to do all the shopping and food preparation, now is an excellent time to break that habit and get others involved. If you live alone, talk to a friend about coordinating shopping so you can help each other out with that quick trip for forgotten items, or offer to share some meal cooking responsibilities.

If you have children, don't forget that they love to help in the kitchen. My son loves to shred veggies in the food processor. It's like running branches through a wood chipper… what could be more fun than that? I do believe that a food processor is a good investment in saving time in the kitchen. It shreds, it creams, it chops, and many of them are now dishwasher safe. But honestly they are not hard to clean. And if you plan ahead you can chop or shred the veggies for the next night's dinner as well and only clean the machine once.

STEP: Figure out the pieces of preparation that can be done by your child, other adults in the house, or members of your community.

Put on some music everyone enjoys and boogie down while you cook. A few extra minutes of preparation time doesn't seem like too much if it's spent working and singing *together* rather than one person hustling to prepare food for those who are begging for dinner to be done.

Question #2) Where is my time wasted when I think I'm actually saving time?

ReCon Your "Convenient" Meal

Baby Steps to Better Health / Baby Step #7

A) How convenient is a convenience stop? Sometimes the kids are melting down and they need something placed right in the pie hole before everyone is a puddle on the floorboards of the car. We've all been there and we have to do something, and it might include fast food or snacks from a convenience store.

Try to stock reasonably healthy snacks in your car for just such occasions. Containers of trail mix made of nuts, dried fruit, & dry cereal keep well and help out when snacks are needed.

Make sure you consider your work and home life when you plan meals, i.e. plan fast meals for nights you need them and longer meals when you have a little more time or someone at home to start the process.

STEP: Time yourself when you make the stop for a convenience meal or a convenience snack, or for a pre-made dinner at the grocery store.

See how long it takes and write it down. So you stop the first place you see and buy some convenience foods. How long does that really take? It depends on where you are, but even if something is close by, you have to park, walk in, choose (with much advice), purchase and go get back in your car, get the food home, unpack it and get it on the table. Time yourself from the minute you deviate from the drive home until people are able to eat.

STEP: Challenge yourself to make a meal, perhaps including leftover grains, or even scrambled eggs and salad in that same amount of time. For extra fun, compare the price of your homemade fast meal to the price of your "convenient" dinner.

Question #3) Where will I find the time that is the difference between pulling something out of the freezer and heating it up and preparing something with real food ingredients from scratch?

Develop a list of quickies.

You might be surprised at the number of recipes out there designed to be ready in 30 minutes or even 20 minutes. There are 2 types of recipes for you to consider:

A) the kind that is actually 20 – 30 minutes from start to finish

B) the kind that is 20 – 30 minutes of prep time but requires some time in between steps for something to boil or roast. These are still possible if you have someone at home who can start that step for you if you are not there. Alternatively, a crock pot or a rice cooker with a built in or old fashioned wall timer can go a long way to help complete some steps by the time you get home.

Baby Steps to Better Health / Baby Step #7

I made stir-fry this evening in 25 minutes and I was not hurrying like I do on nights when one of us is going to an early TaeKwonDo class. I can make pasta from scratch in 30 minutes. It's faster if I sauté double veggies and freeze, that part is done next time around. You can also have a pasta sauce ready at the touch of a blender button, and as fast as the pasta is ready – you can eat (see Easiest Tomato Sauce Ever, p205)!

I made veggie burgers the other day which took a prep time of only about 15 minutes but then they had to bake for 40. I made a bunch, froze the leftovers on the cookie sheet they baked on and now we have a stock of burgers on hand for nights with no time.

STEP: Choose one (or more) night(s) that you are going to try a quick recipe.

Here are a few of our faves: Category A is 20 – 30 minutes until eating, and Category B is 20-30 minutes of prep time with some boiling, roasting or other timed event involved.

A) Anything Goes Fast Burrito(p160);
Pesto Pasta with Veggies and Nuts(p202);
Mushrooms Pignoli(p179);
Noodles with Asian Peanut Sauce(p205);
Varia-Bowl(p207): Category A if using noodles, pasta or leftover grain / Category B if making grains for the meal

B) Herbed Zucchini Rice(p173);
Sushi Salad(p195) (with leftover rice it is in Category A);
Mustard Tempeh(p180) (with leftover rice it is in Category A);
Lentil Casserole(p174)

Wrapping up the Action: Baby Steps for Baby Step #7: Preparing for Healthy Convenience

7-1) Come up with a plan for planning. Or find a source for plans that are already completed, like Little Sis' Weekly Meal Plans.

7-2) Make sure you have containers for holding leftover meals and grains.

7-3) Figure out how to share some shopping and food preparation responsibilities.

7-4) Time yourself when you make the stop for a convenience meal or a convenience snack, or for a pre-made dinner at the grocery store.

7-5) Challenge yourself to make a meal, perhaps including leftover grains, or even scrambled eggs and salad in the same amount of time it took you for step 4.

7-6) Choose one (or more nights) that you are going to try a quick recipe.

Baby Steps to Better Health / Baby Step #7   64.

INSPIRATION:

Remember that one of the most important elements of Baby Steps is that it is okay to make these changes a little at a time. If you eat a healthy fast meal once or twice per week and/or send a healthier lunch once or twice per week more than you do now, then you are improving your health lifestyle. Every day brings new opportunities to make good choices about food. So ReCon commercial convenience…and find ways to have your own healthy convenience instead!

EXPANSION: Plans We Use for Healthy Convenience

So how to manage all this Baby Stepping change? Organization, dear friends, gives me hope! So here is our new plan. We (my husband and I with some input from 11 year old son), plan a week of meals ahead of time. We then make a grocery list, hoping to cut down on trips to the store for the missing ingredients from today's last minute decision for dinner.

We bought these nifty write-on-wipe-off calendar thing-a-ma-bobs, as what is a great plan without needing to buy a thing or two? This helpful thing lives on the fridge.

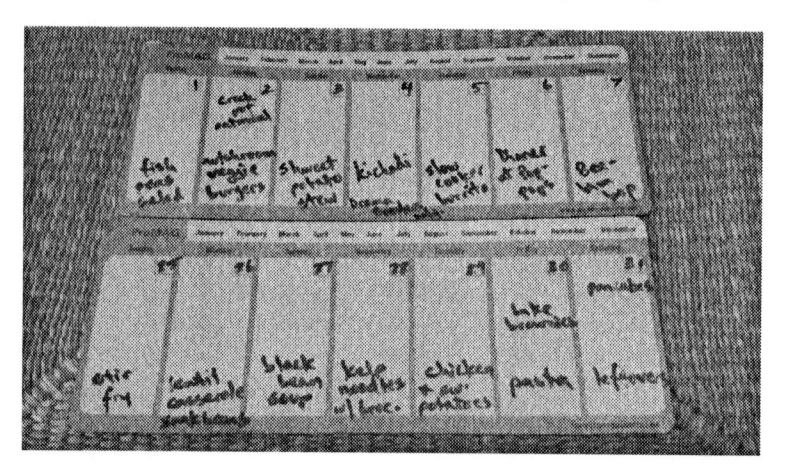

Days I'm working a 12 hour shift, Mr. Bigg Sis (who is generally chief bottle washer and I am chief cook) knows exactly what he is supposed to defrost / prepare / use up, etc. I note when I need to soak beans, nuts or my head on the calendar to forestall the last minute despair over not having soaked almonds for almond milk, or beans for the planned dinner. We include in this plan what our middle schooler will eat for lunch so we can pack it a night or two in advance and take advantage of leftovers.

Other ways we save time in preparing lunch for our growing boy is to pre-pack other parts of the lunch in re-usable containers. We pack fruits in cups, veggies in cups, and snack mixes in cups. We freeze servings of homemade baked goods so we'll have a variety to choose from.

In the morning we heat up and pack the entree in his thermos and choose 1 fruit, 1 veggie, 1 snack mix and 1 baked good to cover lunch and late morning snack in language arts class. My son helps make the snack mixes by choosing trail mix type ingredients that he likes and we mix a variety of: nuts; dried fruit; cereal; popcorn, and crackers into the ever-present plastic cups 10 at a time, again attempting to make more than needed for a while and then he has several mixes to choose from.

Routine is extremely helpful in that the wheel does not need to be re-invented or even re-planned every night. My plan for planning has become a routine that saves us a lot of time and miscommunication.

CHAPTER 8: Baby Step 8 – Change How You Talk and Think About Food

INFORMATION – You listen to yourself.

"Psssst!"

"Who me?"

"Yeah you. The one who is being unkind and intolerant to someone."

"I'm nice to other people, what are you talking about?"

"Everyone?"

"Well, I certainly try."

"And what do you say to yourself when you look in the mirror?"

(silence)

"And what do you say to yourself when you make a mistake or slip up on a plan or intention?"

"Well that doesn't count.... Does it?"

What do you think? Does it count?

When my elementary age students would pronounce themselves stupid or a jerk after making an academic or behavioral mistake, I used to ask them what they would say to their best friend in the same circumstance. They always had lovely encouraging things to say to their best friend. But we don't treat ourselves like a best friend. And although the deep seated human condition from which our self-directed harshness and nastiness arises is beyond my expertise in terms of explanation (or understanding, as I do it too), I do have some suggestions for overcoming it. I believe that a lot of our problems related to diet and food choices stem from negative self-directed language in addition to the language that advertisers greedily drum into our heads.

REFLECTION: Words About Words

A few questions to ask yourself:

> *8a) What do I say inside my head (or out loud) to myself when I make a mistake?*

8b) Do I ever say nice things to myself?

8c) Would I be willing to say nice things to myself?

(Available in Workbook)

It's hard to make choices that value you and your health when you are undermining your own value with your self-directed language.

It's also hard to make choices that value your health when inundated with messages that confuse what it really means to reward yourself.

Would you do the following to someone?
- slap extra pounds on them,
- give diabetes to them,
- add pain to their joints,
- put holes in their teeth,
- burden them with an autoimmune disorder,
- or make them more prone to heart attack or stroke?

Okay, maybe there are a few people in your life that you would curse with the milder choices on the list, however, these things are not rewards. They are punishments. They are also part of life. We don't mean to suggest that everyone who is ill or uncomfortable is being punished or has created that problem for themselves, and we firmly believe that everyone deserves love, respect and help however, changing the way you talk to yourself and think about food could have a huge impact on what you eat and how you feel about yourself and your choices. Your choices can have a huge impact on your actual health and your actual physical experience on the planet. These things in turn can have a huge impact on how you think and feel about yourself – a bit of a circle there. Perhaps our language about food is a good entry point in that cycle. Can changing our words change our choices? We believe that it can.

Baby Step #8 is to pay attention to your language about food. What kind of language do you use to justify poor choices as rewards? How often are your healthy choices described as deprivation? Recognize the language and use it for healthier food. For example, "I have had a hard day at work and I am so tired. I deserve a reward and some TLC. I think I'll eat a big salad and some healthy grains because it will give me energy and take care of my body. I deserve that."

You are not depriving yourself with healthy food. By providing yourself with healthy food you are affirming yourself, because you are valuable and should be treated well. It's internal politics, it's spin doctoring, it's all about attitude baby, and you have some say in how the spin goes down and how the groove is laid in the vinyl. I know I'm dating myself by even mentioning vinyl – but the point is that you can frame your actions in a positive light and make decisions about your language that supports the actions you wish you could take, or that you're trying to take.

When you get to the heart of the matter, food is primarily nourishment. How delightful that it is often also pleasurable and holds such opportunity for fellowship and social interaction. Clearly though food wasn't always, isn't always, and doesn't always have to be pleasurable to the palate… it can be pleasurably nurturing and sustaining to the pancreas, the pulmonary system, the pelvis and the patootie as well. Hungry people eat what is available. Consider that your body is hungry for nutritious food that it recognizes as food. I feel fortunate to have access to clean, healthy, real food. It is possible to find pleasure in providing nourishing food to yourself and you may even find that after a while you prefer the taste of nourishing food. But you have to be on board and that means selling yourself on the program!

ACTION: *Change How You Talk and Think About Food.*

Notice & and write down your language about food.

> *8d) What do you say to yourself before you eat something that you know is not good for you? Is it negative or demeaning to yourself? Is it honest about the food you are about to eat?*
>
> *8e) What do you say before eating something that was not your first impulse choice but that is good for you?*
>
> *8f) Do you expect to like healthy foods?*
>
> *8g) How do you use language about rewards to justify eating unhealthy food?*
>
> *(Available in Workbook)*

2) Substitute positive statements for negative when they happen.

Get past the negative language of deprivation: do not think about NOT having foods you are trying to avoid but about what you are eating instead. A basic tenet of contentment is to give thanks for what you have, rather than long for what you don't have. This can apply to food as well.

Examples:

"I am on a new quest to eat more vegetables and fruits and I am learning all kinds of delicious ways to prepare them."

"How about a delicious fruit & yogurt smoothie for dessert?"

"I feel very fortunate to be able to nourish my body with this healthy food."

I also think it is very helpful to use language that reminds you why you wish to make a healthy food choice as well as language that acknowledges the rewards inherent in good food choices.

"These greens have calcium and iron as well as lots of vitamin A to keep me strong and healthy."

"Real food creates health. I want and deserve good health."

Try using language of rewards in relation to a REAL reward for your body, mind and spirit.

"Real food holds sunshine and soil and water and connects me to this place in a meaningful, fulfilling way."

"I love knowing I'm eating real food."

"I'm going to reward my body with something that is good for it!"

The next step may be especially helpful to your kids, although I also encourage you to voice positive statements like those suggested out loud in front of your kids.

3) Think of someone whose physical abilities you admire and use that admiration to fuel your desire to be healthier.

Think of the physical abilities you would like to have as you eat healthy food that prepares your body to reach its potential. My son wants to be a professional athlete and we discuss that when having disagreements about food choices. We talk about the necessity of taking excellent care of those muscles and bones. It helps him see the value in real food.

4) Link behavior to nutrition.

If you're trying to reduce sugar in a child's diet – explain to them how sugar can affect their health and their behavior. Make sure that you point out to your children what their behavior is like after junk food. They may surprise you by noticing the behavior of their peers and making connections about behavior and food choices. Notice your own

Baby Steps to Better Health / Baby Step #8

behavior and moods in relation to what you eat. Remind yourself, positively, and tell yourself why you are choosing to eat what makes you feel good!

This realization or suggestion can also be a reason to try P.E.P. (pre-emptive produce, i.e. requiring that a piece of fruit or veggie is eaten prior to other snack food) because junk food is less likely to impact behavior when there is something else in the stomach. (The last statement is based on personal experience and observation, not scientific research.) Put something healthy in your stomach first to lessen the amount and impact of eating less healthy stuff. Both of the Sis sisters have noticed that our kids are satisfied with a much smaller quantity of less nutritionally desirable food if they eat something healthful first.

5) Try a non-food or a healthy food reward next time you deserve a treat.

We shared a list of non-food ways to reward yourself in Baby Step #6. I find them very helpful. Experiment with one of our suggestions, or if you haven't already, create your own list of non-food rewards.

Wrapping up the Action: Baby Steps for Baby Step #8: Change How You Talk and Think About Food

8-1) Notice (and write down) your language about food.

8-2) Substitute positive statements for negative when they happen.

8-3) Think of someone whose physical abilities you admire and use that admiration to fuel your desire to be healthier.

8-4) Link behavior to nutrition.

8-5) Try a non-food or a healthy food reward next time you deserve or need a treat.

(Available in Workbook)

INSPIRATION:

This culture of 'treating' ourselves in detrimental ways is pervasive, even appearing at schools, but if you make the language involved you use about food more honest, you might have more luck overcoming it! Using positive language is generally more engaging with others and perhaps you will get farther changing the culture at the places you gather and spend time to include healthy choices for mealtimes and snack times.

Remember that Baby Steps mean a bit of change at a time and an endless supply of second chances. Pay attention to your language about food. It affects what you eat,

Baby Steps to Better Health / Baby Step #8   71.

how you feel about what you eat, and your health. Pay attention to your language about yourself. It affects who you are, how you feel about who you are, and your health!

Does this sound plausible to you? "I am really upset about _____ and I need something to make me feel better. I'm going to make a cup of tea and call my best friend. Or I'm just going to say to myself what I know she would say to me if she were here." (What would my wonderful Sis say for instance.) I have a pretty good & comforting guess… and it's a lot better than what I'd say to myself most of the time.

You are valuable. You are loved. You are worthy and your body wants to serve you. You deserve to eat real food.

EXPANSION:

If you would like to further explore the idea that how you talk to yourself can have an impact on your behavior and your attitude, try doing a search on the terms, "self-talk", "you are what you say", and "power of positive thinking."

You can also ponder Little Sis' thoughts on how we think about and talk to ourselves about food:

"Minding the Gap"

You never know what will prompt a realization about food, patterns and change. I had a mini-revelation about my own eating evolution while completing a home improvement project this week, and if you'll indulge me, I'd like to share that with you.

Our back door has never really closed properly. The lock stuck, the handle was dodgy, and worst of all, there was a visible gap when the door was closed. I could see light coming in. And if there's light, there is a draft I must stamp out. I HATE drafts. The well-installed door jamb insulation just didn't seem to cut the mustard. Because we had no idea what we were doing and because we had some on hand, we stuffed some rubber insulating crap into the gap. The kind that sticks on one side and sits in the gap when the door is closed. It blocked the draft, for a while. In case you're wondering, we will get to food.

You know what happens with sticky stuff exposed to cold. It doesn't stick for long, especially if it is in an area that is frequently touched by twin outdoor enthusiasts. One layer of rubber insulating crap out, another in. After some consideration, we did the only logical thing and replaced the rubber crap with a metal strip that was nailed into the jam. It stayed there good. It closed some of the gap, and increased the effort required to close and lock the door significantly. And there was still light coming in. You know what we did? We jammed some more crap in there. And every morning when the dog was let out, and the crap fell, we re-inserted it to keep the draft out. It worked, well sort of, if you got it in there just right EVERY time, and the dog didn't run off with some of the sticky rubber attached to his back, and you threw the door closed with your hips so you could turn the lock; three layers of crap really ought to work, and yet I knew it was all wrong. Worst of all, I was still cold. In case you're wondering, we will get to food.

A few minutes on YouTube (ain't the internet grand?) and I knew that I had taken the wrong approach from the outset. I didn't need to fill the gap. I needed to mind it. I needed to address the daggone gap. Reviewed YouTube video, grabbed screwdriver, utility knife, and my favorite mini pry bar. I systematically took all the crap out of the gap (except for the initial bit of professionally-installed weather stripping at the edge of the jamb). A few nail holes that can be painted over (when the enthusiasm for that erupts) were all that remained. I then removed the strike plates (thanks YouTube for the lingo) and moved them closer to the outside of the house, dug out the latch and lock holes with the utility knife. I made the gap smaller. Guess what happened? I closed the door easily, locked it with no trouble and was greeted by a dark door jamb, nary a ray of light, and no moving air. Hallelujah.

The funny part is, and I appreciate your sticking with me to see how this has anything to do with Baby Steps to Better Health, I couldn't help but see this relatively simple (albeit long overdue) home repair as the perfect analogy for the relationship that so many of us have with food. We know that the food that we eat is not necessarily nourishing; we believe we should do better. We feel the draft and sense that the choices that we are making are not helping us feel our best, but like my home improvement project, we fail to look at the root long enough to address the problem. Instead of minding the gap between what we know or think we probably should do and what we are in fact doing, we stuff in a bunch of crap.

Sometimes it's literal, we stuff in a bunch of junk food because it's a fast fix to hunger and we don't have time to think about doing more. We stuff in diet food because we want to manage our weight and are unsure of how to do that on our own. We stuff in the food that is so readily available and that we've been led to believe is making our life easier. Like my rubber weather stripping, the crap doesn't stick and just creates a whole new set of problems. The gap persists, and in fact widens each time we stuff crap in. In my own relationship with food, I got so good at filling the gap with crap that I ultimately chose the material that can fill a gap in the most destructive way. Guilt.

Rather than addressing the root of the problem I simply continued with my habits, but I was sure to feel guilty about it. If I was really on a roll, I'd make fun of myself. "Wow, look at that nutritious meal. Definitely not having a heart attack after this. That'll help the pants fit better." Wasn't I funny? And so unhappy and chilled by the draft. I sat there, judged myself, found myself wanting, and then did everything I could to make it worse. It took me a VERY long time to mind the gap. Why aren't I taking better care of myself? Why aren't I at least making easy switches that I'm told would improve my

Baby Steps to Better Health / Baby Step #8

health? Why am I rolling my eyes at my sister who is trying to help me instead of at least listening with an open mind?

The way to feel better, for me, was to make the gap smaller. I needed to make the gap between healthy choices and the lifestyle I was actually living smaller. Avoiding the problem, replacing favorite foods with diet versions of favorite foods, and feeling guilty all worked together to sink my body image and land me in a nasty bit of a hole. A cold, drafty depressing hole. The only way to solve the problem was to mind the gap, and then to decide to make it smaller.

If you know you've got a gap, and you feel the draft, or if you're stuffing crap in the draft, maybe today is your day. Maybe today is the day to mind the gap, and make it just the slightest bit smaller. A little baby step smaller. We're here to help, to cheer you on, and to give you some food choices that won't leave you cold. Maybe our super easy lentil casserole, or a simple stir fry would be good places to take a little step. Maybe you want to add some veggies (or at least know you need to) – how about some crowd pleasing green beans? Maybe sweets are your downfall…. Check out the Desserts & Sweets section(p143) in the recipes at the back for some lower sugar snacks. Mind the gap. You'll be glad you did.

CHAPTER 9: Baby Step 9 – How to Replace Processed Foods with Real Foods

INFORMATION: You can step up to the (new) plate.

In the interest of clarity and ease, we thought we'd take a departure from our usual path and make some specific suggestions of how to baby step down on some highly processed foods that are 1) full of junk you don't want to eat and 2) empty of real nourishment for that beautiful bod. These are meant as examples, although if you wanted to get started on these specific changes right here today, I could hardly fault you for your enthusiasm ;-). You may feel like you can skip this chapter, and that's okay as well.

REFLECTION: It's an ongoing but worthwhile battle.

The folks that make processed food know what makes us want more. The advertising folks they hire know what makes us want to try, buy and NEVER deny. It's an ongoing battle for your health. Think about what drives you to choose processed food. Know where the battle is hardest for you.

> *9a) What occasions/ days are full of processed food in my life?*
>
> *9b) Am I adding the processed food to my (our) diet or is someone(thing) else (like a relative, friend, or tradition)?*
>
> *9c) When my celebrations include processed food, what else could I do to celebrate?*
>
> *(Available in Workbook)*

ACTION: Back away from the processed foods slowly with your hands up.

I. Our first candidate for baby stepping is quintessential Americana, and I'll bet many of you have a version you just love: macaroni and cheese. Now, please understand me, I have long been a fan of the macaroni noodle and I see no reason why it and something creamy and salty shouldn't be consumed often and with great gusto, but the boxed 'convenience food' version of this modern day miracle is a pale reflection of the food that could be on your plate. So let's begin with this convenient and inexpensive little box beloved by kids and parents alike for the ease of pleasing. Truth is those boxes contain Yellow #5 and Yellow #6 which the Center for Science in the Public Interest (CSPI) says we should AVOID EATING ("unsafe in amounts consumed or very poorly tested and not worth any risk").[30] These boxes contain all manner of other things like MSG that are also considered wise to restrict and or avoid. The convenience comes at a price, apparently.

If you start with Kraft (or one of its many generic clones) Macaroni and Cheese your steps could look like this:

Step 1) a boxed mac n cheese that boasts fewer artificial colors and preservatives (which you will use less often because they are, admittedly, more expensive)

Step 2) easy homemade mac n cheese (Instantly Healthier Mac & Cheese(p174) made with white noodles and cheddar cheese

Step 3) a natural boxed mac n cheese that uses whole grain noodles and cheddar cheese (again more costly)

Step 4) easy homemade mac n cheese made with whole grain noodles (why whole grain? – see expansion section) – Instantly Healthier Mac & Cheese without the Box (p174)

Step 5) homemade mac n cheese with whole grain noodles and added veggies (maybe a crumb topping will engage a few more people) – see our Zucheezy Noodles(p202)

The Bonus Round? Ditch the pasta (and yes, it pains me to say that) in favor of a whole grain (see Baby Step # 3b, or the expansion section of this chapter for suggestions on how to cook them) with whatever passes for cheese or creaminess for you and, of course, first and foremost, keep those veggies.

Ta Da!! You've ended with a meal that is lower in sugar, preservatives, and artificial colorings, boasts the nutritional value of included veggies and whole grains and lacks stuff of dubious and unknown origins. The really delightful thing is that the homemade versions will also provide you with excellent bang for your buck, particularly as the nutritional content increases. People who are getting what they need from food don't tend to need to eat as much of it – at least that's been my experience. You may also find, after all of that baby stepping, that making your own version of this processed favorite really doesn't take that long. My son could make our healthy, homemade 'Instant' Mac & Cheese when he was 10. On to the next hill!

II. Our second candidate for baby stepping down is a staple (and has been a staple) for so many people for so very long – the staff of life they call it. Truthfully though, the bread that you can buy in the store today bears little resemblance to bread that people have relied upon around the world for centuries. A lot of commercially prepared bread contains high fructose corn syrup (which our friends over at CSPI agree we should all cut back on).[31] There is a substantial list of long chemical names at the end of many of these ingredient lists that I simply don't understand and dismiss as being unnecessary having made bread many times. The other neat thing about the label on white bread is that the flour that it contains is "enriched." They've added some vitamins and minerals back in. They put them in there because the process that they put the grain through to make it into fluffy white flour takes it all out – everything. The process removes all that is nutritious beyond the benefit of pure calories, which most of us are not lacking! Personally, I'm not convinced that throwing some riboflavin in there is going make up for the difference, but I might be a little cynical that way. You CAN have the convenience of bread but get more out of it nutritionally by stepping up to bread that packs a punch for your body.

If you start with Wonder (or one of its many white bread clones out there), your steps could look something like this:

Step 1) a loaf of wheat bread (I mean the brown stuff. I suggest going for the brown stuff right off the bat, but get the super soft stuff that is shaped as much like your regular loaf as possible. This is the big step on this one, IMO. There are folks who really struggle to get past the color of wheat bread. If you and yours can make this switch, the rest of these steps are pretty smooth sailing.),

Step 2) a loaf of wheat bread that specifically lists *whole* wheat in the ingredients list,

Step 3) a loaf of wheat bread that is described on its main label as "whole wheat bread",

Step 4) a loaf of whole wheat bread that has at least 3 grams of fiber per slice,

Step 5) a loaf of 100% whole wheat bread,

Step 6) a loaf of 100% whole wheat bread that doesn't contain high fructose corn syrup,

Bonus Round: sprouted wheat bread OR homemade 100% whole wheat or whole grain bread.

Ta Dah! Now a sandwich is more than cellulose fiber, empty calories and whatever you put in the middle. Let's keep trucking…

III. Non-Dairy Coffee Creamer. If you are anywhere near my age, long ago you saw a movie called "Say Anything". My favorite line in this movie is delivered by older sister to the ever popular Lloyd Doebler in response to what she understands that he has eaten for the day: "There's no food in your food." If there ever was a food product for which this line is a perfect description, it is non-dairy coffee creamer. I should admit that I am suspicious of any product that is sold to me largely by what it is not rather than what it is: "non-dairy" "non-fat" "low-fat." That's all well and good, but WHAT IS IT?! Well, I'll tell you. It's corn syrup solids, partially hydrogenated soybean oil,

Baby Steps to Better Health / Baby Step #9

sodium caseinate, artificial colors and artificial flavors… and that's for the unflavored variety. There is no food in that food.

Don't get me wrong, I can appreciate a good doctored up coffee; I worked at a coffee bar BEFORE barristas people. I understand we do not all enjoy the dark power of that hot bitter cup of morning life (yes, I have a problem), but let's not just go putting any old thing in there, shall we?

If you start with a flavored non-dairy creamer type thing….here's how to back away with your healthy hands up.

Step 1) Try cream or half and half and some hot cocoa mix or chocolate syrup (these often also have chemicals but if you are mixing you at least have control over the amount).

Step 2) How about milk (or nut milk) and some straight up sugar? Again, you can control that amount and baby step it down over time.

Step 3) How about milk (or nut milk) and some maple syrup (it is good, I swear). Cinnamon is a nice flavor as well – and it lends a little sweetness.

Step 4) How about just plain milk (or nut milk)?

Bonus Round: switch out a cup of whatever kind of coffee you're drinking for green tea and have a glass of water in the morning when you wake up BEFORE you pour that cuppa joe.

Ta Dah! There is now more food in your food. You can now pursue your lifelong dream of being a professional kick boxer, sport of the future you know.

INSPIRATION: We all struggle with food choices. Inspire yourself with the words, thoughts or actions of others.

Here are some quotes on eating that may inspire you. I found these as part of a poster for free download at the site of a psychologist named Dr. Susan Albers[32] who writes books about mindful eating and explores the emotional component of eating.

"One cannot think well, love well, sleep well, if one has not dined well." - Virginia Woolf

"Let food be thy medicine, thy medicine shall be thy food." - Hippocrates

"Tell me what you eat and I will tell you who you are." - Brillat-Savarin

Baby Steps to Better Health / Baby Step #9

"The doctor of the future will give no medication, but will interest his patients in the care of the human frame, diet, and in the cause and prevention of disease." - Thomas Edison

EXPANSION: *Why whole grain and Why switch my pasta for a grain?*

1) Why whole grain?

Semolina pasta (the kind most folks are accustomed to and that you find the most of at the store) is made from enriched grain. Basically, enriched grain is processed grain that has vitamins and/or minerals added back to it after most of the nutrients are removed during the processing, which removes parts of the grain like the hull. Unfortunately it is impossible to put everything back in. We don't know everything that is valuable in plants, we haven't isolated it all and therefore can't put it back. Where would the processor get it from if they could? The pile of stuff they just took out, right? We know some vitamins and minerals to replace and that's what is added back into enriched grains, but there are arguments that supplement versions of vitamins and minerals are not as beneficial as what is found in plants and animals, i.e. whole food.[33] In addition, during grain processing, fiber is removed with the hull. Why not just leave it all in there and eat the whole healthy she-bang? I mean she-grain?

You don't have to listen to me when you can listen to the Harvard School of Public Health:
"A growing body of research shows that returning to whole grains and other less-processed sources of carbohydrates and cutting back on refined grains improves health in myriad ways. As researchers have begun to look more closely at carbohydrates and health, they are learning that the quality of the carbohydrates you eat is at least as important as the quantity. Most studies, including some from several different Harvard teams, show a connection between eating whole grains and better health."[34]

The article summarizes many benefits of eating whole grains including:
• Benefits to the cardiovascular system via lowering total cholesterol and reduced risk of heart attack, stroke or the need for heart surgery;
• Decreased risk of developing Type 2 Diabetes ("Researchers estimate that swapping whole grains in place of even some white rice could lower diabetes risk by 36 percent."[35] That sounds like a Baby Step to me!);
• Possible protection against cancer;
• Prevention of constipation and diverticular disease; and
• Decrease in other risks for death from inflammation-related, noncardiac, noncancer causes.

Baby Steps to Better Health / Baby Step #9

2) Comparison of white and wheat pasta:

Nutritionist Joy Bauer explains the benefits of whole wheat pasta: "A 100 percent whole-grain pasta includes all three layers of the wheat kernel: the bran, the germ and the endosperm. Because nothing is removed during processing, whole-grain pastas contain more natural fiber and micronutrients than their white, refined cousins. And thanks to the extra fiber, whole-grain pastas tend to be more filling than traditional white pasta. What's more, regularly choosing whole-grains over the refined type is associated with numerous health benefits, including lower blood pressure and reduced risk of many chronic diseases, including type 2 diabetes and heart disease. " BIG BABY STEP MOMENT HERE, FRIENDS. If you still eat semolina pasta, give whole wheat a try. If you are skeptical, start with a blended pasta. These have more whole grains than straight semolina, but less than 100% whole grain pasta. Take the pasta dish your family enjoys the most, and make a relatively small change that can add up to big benefits.

I have on my lap two packages of dried pasta. One is 100% whole wheat chicciole (giant puffy elbows), the other is 100% semolina ziti (purchased for necklace production last summer). Let's compare the nutrition low-down. Nutritional info is based on a two ounce serving in both cases.

100% Whole Wheat	100% Semolina
Calories: 180	Calories: 210
Total Fat: 1.5g	Total Fat: 1g
Total Carbohydrate: 35g	Total Carbohydrate: 42g
Dietary Fiber: 6g	Dietary Fiber: 2g
Sugars: 1g	Sugars: 3g
Protein: 7g	Protein: 7g

The Sis sisters LOVE pasta and there are many pasta dishes in our recipes section.

3) Why would I switch out my pasta for a grain?

It's a matter of variety you spicy thing you! Pasta made from whole grain wheat has certain nutrients; grains like brown rice, quinoa, barley, steel cut oats, buckwheat, kamut, wild rice and millet have other nutrients – and other flavors. If you can put it on pasta, you can probably put it on a grain! Some grains will not require as much sauce / topping / vegetables as you might like on pasta, so add some, taste and add some more, but give whole grains a try!

Here are some grain recipes to check out in the Recipe section:
Cool Summer Veggie Quinoa(p211)
Power Tabbouleh(p186)
Herbed Sweet Tomatoes with Rice(p215)

And here are some pasta dishes to try over whole grain pasta or grains:
Walnut Pesto(p202)
Whole Wheat Bowties with Roasted Cauliflower(p222)
Easiest Tomato Sauce Ever(p205)

CHAPTER 10: Baby Step #10: Understanding the Importance of Amount

INFORMATION: Less IS less and More IS more.

My Southern grandmother's way of asking if we wanted more food was not, "Would you like some more?" It was "What'll you have?"

In other words, "Which of these delicious things will you have more of now?" And it was hard, both physically and socially, to not promptly pick your personal favorite of her offerings. For me it was her hot milk cake, her watermelon rind pickles, her homemade biscuits with homemade plum jelly or her sugar cookies. Notice the sweet theme… oh yes, I was a sugar hound!! It was not only personally satisfying but socially satisfying to have more.

Our culture has become very much about more. If you haven't seen the film Super Size Me, I highly recommend it for an eye opener on serving sizes in fast food restaurants. The film has some rough language and frank talk about sex, (and the effects bad food can have on sexual desire and performance), so may not be appropriate for younger kids. The movie highlights the growth in serving sizes and some fast food restaurants have responded by eliminating their largest "super" sizes. The fact remains, however, that even their small offerings are far larger than they have been at times in the past. Many restaurant servings far exceed recommended serving sizes and all of these big foods affect not just our health, but our perceptions about what a normal portion looks like.[36]

Check out how portions have increased over the years[37] (and this includes the size of plates!).[38]

	Portion / Calories 20 years ago	Portion / Calories Today
Bagel	3" diameter / 140 cal.	6" diameter / 350
Cheeseburger	1 / 333 cal.	1 / 590 cal.
Spaghetti w/ meatballs	1 cup sauce 3 small meatballs / 500 cal.	2 cups sauce 3 large meatballs / 1,020 cal.
Soda	6.5 ounces / 82 cal.	20 ounces / 250 cal.
Blueberry Muffin	1.5 ounces / 210 cal.	5 ounces / 500 cal.

REFLECTION: *The message on eating is usually the more the merrier, the bigger the better!*

While our portion sizes have increased, we continue to be surrounded with images and messages that indicate that we should have little bitty skinny bodies (with very large breasts), and that we should make up for that difference with a sparkling new (and expensive) gym membership, and/or trip to the plastic surgeon. It would seem that we are in a watermelon rind pickle indeed. And apparently, it's a much larger watermelon rind pickle than I ate as a child.

Of course, weight is not the only issue of concern, but to be honest, it is often the issue that leads people to change their game. It certainly played a role in my desire to eat more healthfully. Even so, controlling weight and embracing good health is about so much more than food. That's why it is so difficult. Even Oprah Winfrey, who can hire the best chefs in the world to prepare spectacularly delicious healthy food, struggles with her weight. Food is so much more than nourishment to us. As givers and recipients of food we have a lot to sort through when it comes to food choices and the health effects we generate.

People will argue over whether *what* you eat, or *how much* you eat has a greater impact on health and weight. Of course, as is so often the case when it comes to factors that affect our health, paying attention to both makes a lot of sense. We have talked a lot in our Baby Steps series about *what* you eat. We should put a little attention here on *how much* you eat. Buckle up because American advertising and culture has set us up for a fall here.

Let me illustrate with an example. As a teenager we had a Farrells' Ice Cream Parlor in our town. Farrell's offered a ridiculously large banana split and a promise. If you finished the ridiculously large banana split, you got a button that said, "I made a pig of myself at Farrell's!" The button was delivered by servers who were banging a drum and making a big, entertaining fuss out of you... the pig... for finishing the ridiculously large dish of ice cream. These buttons were worn with pride. I'm sure you've encountered similar contests at other restaurants. Big Bro (not to be confused with Biggest Bro of sneezing-on-his-French-Fries-to-prevent-theft fame) once won a pie eating contest. His prize was a coupon for a free cheeseburger and fries at a local deli. He almost threw up when they announced his prize.

It is not simply that our serving sizes have become too large, but that we celebrate our overeating... we revel in it. We feel that we are getting a prize, or more often a REALLY good deal, when we get the cup of brown fizz that's large enough to bathe in. The opportunities to consume large portions are everywhere, and food purveyors want you to feel good about that. You will be even more awesome if you eat that whole pie, that whole banana split, or that whole extra "value" meal.

Baby Steps to Better Health / Baby Step #10   83.

> *10a) How do you decide how much to eat?*
>
> *10b) Do you limit your number of servings?*
>
> *10c) Does the amount of food vary depending on how active you were that day?*
>
> *10d) Are the bowls and plates you use bigger than those you used to use or used as a child?*
>
> *(Available in Workbook)*

ACTION: Understanding the Importance of Amount

There are a few tricks to eating less and one of them is to understand what a reasonable portion is. Knowledge is power, right? I think that this is one of the reasons why Weight Watchers is one of the few truly successful weight loss programs out there. They teach portion control. So, here are some tips for eating less…. eating less bad stuff…. and finally in the Expansion section some comparisons of food serving size to everyday objects to help your eyes and brain become accustomed to reasonable food portions.

1) Start with vegetables. It is not possible to eat too many vegetables, unless they are deep fried. Really. I don't recommend consuming a whole bag of greens in one setting as you might be asking for a little digestive trouble, but seriously, you will know when you've had enough vegetables. Get your stomach a little full with vegetables. Use Pre-emptive Produce (PEP). We talked about this once before… but it can be used at mealtimes as well as at snacktime. Before a snack of the salty or sweet variety can take place, a serving of fruit or vegetable must happen. Thus, my son eats a carrot or a half an apple before he can have some pretzels or a cookie after school. Likewise, eating your veggies first at mealtime – and slipping in more is even better – leaves less room for the other things on your plate.

2) Slow down. Lots of research shows that the hormones that indicate satiation take a little while to let us know we are full. That's why sometimes you don't get uncomfortably full until a little after you eat. You were full before you stopped, you just didn't know it yet.

3) Use smaller plates. This is a restaurant trick and it works very well. A serving looks smaller on a large plate and larger on a small plate. Choose the smaller plate or bowl and then your eyes will be closer to the size of your stomach. Little Sis and her family

Baby Steps to Better Health / Baby Step #10

routinely eat their meals on salad plates. It's much easier to serve yourself a reasonable amount of food when you don't have all that blank plate to stare at.

4) When snacking – Put your snack into a small dish and then put the bag / container away before taking the dish to the couch or your desk or out on the deck. It is nearly impossible to practice portion control with a whole box, bag or container of something you enjoy right in front of you.

5) Make extra of your favorite vegetable dishes and use them as a snack. We've been taught that a snack means a handful of unhealthy items. Buck that trend and eat some roasted potatoes, sweet potatoes and beets, or creamed kale or special green beans. You'll be glad you did. And again – when was the last time somebody ate a whole container of vegetables? A whole bag of potato chips? A whole bag of oreos? An entire bunch of broccoli?

6) Share an entree at a restaurant with someone. You might be pleasantly surprised by how full you are for less money! Also consider ordering an appetizer as your main event. Appetizers are smaller, less expensive, and more often than not, the yummiest part of the menu.

7) Allow yourself to sense the pleasure the food brings (i.e. really pay attention to the act of eating). How can you feel satiated or really enjoy that wonderful taste, creaminess, crunchiness, or whatever your flavor might be, if you are not even noticing it? Are you eating while watching TV, studying, playing on your phone or reading? Or are you actually paying attention to the pleasure of the reasonable portion that you placed in a bowl and are enjoying after eating a piece of PEP?

Paying attention to our food is a recurrent them that we've addressed in previous steps by writing down what we are eating, looking at our pantries; and thinking about why we eat what we eat. Putting your attention on how much you eat: reading labels to notice the recommended serving size; paying attention to the size of your plate or bowl; and knowing that you might just feel full if you take a breather for about 20 minutes will help you control your portions.

Wrapping Up the Action: Baby Steps for Baby Step #10: Understanding the Importance of Amount

10-1) Choose 2 of these portion control strategies to try this week

10-2) Choose 2 more to try next week

10-3) Or set your own pace to try these tricks, but choose the strategies you will try.

Baby Steps to Better Health / Baby Step #10

10-4) Cut yourself a break and try again if you don't make it. Remember that you are in control of your own plan here; small goals, small steps, big successes, and another baby step to better health!

(Available in Workbook)

INSPIRATION: Are you satisfied?

Little Sis has a question she uses at the dinner table with her children when they are stating that they are done. Admittedly this question is only asked after some sort of vegetable matter has been consumed, however it is an important question for all of us to ask ourselves.

"Mama, may I be excused?"
"Are you satisfied?"

Are you satisfied? This is of course a question with many, many layers, but one which can help us all tackle our learned and innate desire to have a lot. You CAN stop eating when you are satisfied but it is much easier to do that if you acknowledge that you are indeed satisfied as far as food is concerned. You are not trying to gauge if you are FULL, which is to say that you couldn't eat any more without being truly uncomfortable. You are determining whether or not your hunger has been satisfied. - Are you no longer hungry? Feeling like you've been re-fueled? Have you supplied your body with what it needs? If you have satisfied your need for food and you are still not satisfied, then perhaps some thoughts about other ways than food to satisfy yourself are in order. Perhaps you need some human contact? Perhaps you need a purpose? Perhaps you need some spiritual guidance? I am not trying to be flippant. The question "Are you satisfied?" can reveal some deep needs while it allows us to stop eating, because truly, food of any sort can only fill some of the longings and needs that we have. You deserve to explore all of the avenues of your life.... all of the faculties and longings of mind, body and spirit that make you human and hold such potential for personal and communal satisfaction.

EXPANSION: Portion Size

The University of California at Berkeley makes some comparisons between household objects and measurements of food to help you visualize just what constitutes the serving size listed on the nutrition labels.[39]

Grains: A serving of grains is like a half of a modern bagel (remember they used to be smaller!!) or an adult fist is about 1 cup of rice, pasta or cereal.

Fruits / Veggies: A serving of fruit or veggie is one about the size of a tennis ball. A cup of salad is about the amount you could hold in your cupped hands (but I wouldn't worry about how much salad you eat - it's the dressing and the potato salad and the macaroni salad that you add that will make salad a portion or weight problem).

Dairy: An ounce of cheese is about the size of 4 playing dice. If you know the size of your yogurt cup, then you have an idea of about 6 oz or 8 oz of liquid or creamy type foods. (Watch your yogurt labels however for the incredible amount of sugar!)

Meat: A 3 oz. serving of meat, poultry or fish is about the size of a deck of cards. 2 Tablespoons of peanut butter is about the size of a golf ball.

Oils: A teaspoon of butter is 1/3rd of the Tablespoon marking on the side of most sticks of butter or about the size of 2 stacked nickels. I suggest you go ahead and measure a teaspoon or 2 of dressing or oil before you place it on your next salad and see how much is there!

Be particularly aware of sweetened beverage sizes. Sweetened beverages used to be a treat, not the staple daily source of hydration. People drank water and milk with small glasses of juice or soda here and there and those portions were more like 4 – 8 ounces; even my sweet treat providing grandmother served Coca Cola in a juice glass – with ice in it. A juice glass is a far cry from the 20oz sodas often found in vending machines or the 30oz. of a Big Gulp. I know for a fact that people who buy a Big Gulp on the way to work could not possibly be a nurse because nurses don't get enough breaks in the day for a Big Urinate! Sweetened beverages are a great target for Baby Step #1, if you haven't already tackled them.

CHAPTER 11: Baby Step 11 – Finding and Doling out the Food Dollars: You Can Afford Healthy Food

INFORMATION: There are hidden costs to poor food choices.

While Little Sis and I have created some cheap healthy recipes (a list is in the expansion section), and can make many things ourselves more cheaply than we can buy them (almond milk, almond butter, high quality baked goods, macaroni & cheese, salad dressing, etc.), there is no denying that fresh fruits and vegetables, especially organic ones, cost more than a cart full of hamburger helper and canned green beans. However, the comparison is not fair unless you consider the entire picture of food costs. In order to accurately consider food costs you must consider cost per nutrient, cost per week or month rather than 1 meal, and the cost of healthcare associated with some cheap but unhealthy foods.

REFLECTION: What does your food... all of your food, really cost?

Time and cost are the two main barriers for people in improving their diet with healthy or real food (like produce, whole grains, or organic meat). We tackled the problem of time spent preparing healthier foods in Baby Step # 7, so it's time to focus on the argument that it costs too much to eat healthier food.

Food is available in many places, almost every place these days, and prices do vary. I'm sure you've noticed. It always hurts me to pay twice or three times as much for a granola bar in a convenience store than I would have paid had I bought a box at the grocery store, or made a snack ahead of time and brought it along.

It also hurts me to pay for food at work that costs much more than it would have cost me to pack leftovers because I ran out of time, or left my lunch at home. We all turn to these expensive conveniences from time to time, but we can't honestly assess what we are spending on food each week or each month if we don't include our expenditures outside of the grocery store. I confess that my grocery bills are higher since we have begun eating more real food (un-prepared, un-processed fresh and some frozen foods). However, I also spend less in restaurants, convenience stores, at work, or on outings than I did previous to the change in diet.

> *11a) Are there times when you are caught without food for yourself or your children – be it a meal or a snack? What do you do?*
>
> *11b) Are there nights or times when someone or the whole family eats out because it is more convenient?*

11c) Is your use of restaurants planned into your budget?

(Available in Workbook)

A true comparison of the cost of healthy vs. unhealthy eating goes beyond an accurate tally of all the money we spend on food, both in and out of the grocery store. A true and fair comparison of costs includes information about the food eaten and its impact on your body.

We will consider 3 ways to compare the cost of food:

A) Cost per nutrient: How much food is in your food?

B) Cost per week or month: How much are you REALLY spending on food?

C) Cost considering long term cost of healthcare / ill health: What will your food choices cost you in the long run?

A) How much food is in your food?

When you pay $1 for a box of cheap macaroni & cheese what are you getting? You are getting calories but not a lot of nutrition. Some would argue that we might even eat more when we eat poorly (from a nutritional standpoint) because our bodies send us messages to eat more in search of missing nutrients.

A USDA report (2012),[40] found that healthy foods are actually cheaper than processed foods when viewed from a nutritional rather than a caloric standpoint. If food is just to be fuel, all you need are calories – you will be able to "keep going." But if you want the machine that is your beautiful body to feel good, to perform well, to fight off all the germies floating around… well then your beautiful machine needs more than calories. The body requires a variety of nutrients - all those complex bits that get stripped out, and occasionally stuffed back in limited numbers into processed foods. The body hungers for nutrition, not just calories. When you buy real foods, you get those nutrients and the money you've spent actually buys you more than just enough fuel to trudge along.

There are many benefits to providing the body with nutrition rather than just fuel. The Mayo Clinic's website[41] discusses a study that showed that children who eat 'slow food' (versus fast food) have more cognitive gains and growth. It is a full-brainer to eat healthy food!

You just might find that you feel 'more full' after eating real food…. and less tempted to have seconds, or dessert, or a large serving of chips later in the evening. Satiation is important to stopping eating. Doesn't it make sense that your body will be more satiated by foods that actually deliver nutrients?

Baby Steps to Better Health / Baby Step #11

B) How much are you REALLY spending on food?

Do you only consider what you spend at the grocery store to be what you spend on food? When I say grocery store it is a short way of saying planned primary food purchasing. You may also use a farmers market, a CSA (Consumer Sponsored Agriculture)[42] or buy chickens or eggs from a friend or neighbor. All of that procurement of food to be stored, prepared and/or consumed in your home is your expected food expenditure and perhaps what you include in your weekly or monthly budget for food.

But that's not the whole food budget story, is it? You likely spend money on food or beverages at coffee shops, vending machines, convenience stores, ball games or other sporting events or school events. Money spent at restaurants is also part of your total food expenditure. We are not suggesting here that any of these expenditures are inherently bad, however, in order to have a complete picture of your food budget and to compare it to the cost of eating more healthfully, you must include all of money that you spend on food – restaurant food, unplanned convenience food, snacks, and treats.

C) What will your food choices cost you in the long run?

"Who would have thought you could fight cancer, diabetes, heart disease and stroke … with a fork? Many people don't know it, but one of the most important things you can do to protect yourself from these diseases is to eat a healthy diet"[43] (Everyday Choices, 2011 - a joint effort of the American Cancer Society, the American Diabetes Association and the American Heart Association). Of course nobody wants any of these diseases, but any perceived barriers to eating well might also be barriers to a healthier future. Within our comparison of the cost of healthy (real) food versus unhealthy (processed) food, it makes sense to consider current and future healthcare costs.

While there is always the chance of a broken leg or a bad case of the flu to increase your healthcare costs, the above warning regarding cancer, heart disease and diabetes warrants a deeper look. As of 2010, the Centers for Disease Control (CDC) estimated that 25.8 million people, or 8.3% of the U.S. population, have diabetes.[44] "People with diagnosed diabetes incur average medical expenditures of about $13,700 per year, of which about $7,900 is attributed to diabetes. People with diagnosed diabetes, on average, have medical expenditures approximately 2.3 times higher than what expenditures would be in the absence of diabetes"[45] (American Diabetes Association, 2013). Diabetes definitely carries financial as well as physical burdens. The good news is that Type II Diabetes represents 90 – 95% of all cases of diabetes[46] and is a preventable disease. Type II Diabetes can be prevented through healthy choices.

This is just one example of the effect that a preventable disease can have on your healthcare expenditures. The money you spend on real food now can have a positive effect on what you will have to spend to maintain the longevity and quality of life that we all desire as we age.

> **11d) Do you read nutrition labels? Does your meal planning ensure the inclusion of fruits and/or vegetables in each meal?**
>
> **11e) Do you have a system to keep track of money spent on food that is not the grocery store / farmer's market?**
>
> **11f) Is your use of restaurants planned into your budget?**
>
> **11g) Are you spending money to treat a disease that could be improved with diet?**
>
> *(Available in Workbook)*

ACTION: *Understanding the Importance of Amount.*

Now that you've thought about the hidden costs of food, you are better equipped to make a fair comparison and decide whether or not you can afford to eat more healthy (real) food in place of unhealthy (processed) food.

A) Cost per nutrients: How much food is in your food?

Baby Step Action: Pay attention to what foods you buy – not just from a cost perspective, but from a nutritional standpoint as well. Consider the nutritive value when you purchase a packet of whole grain pasta versus white pasta or a box of hamburger helper versus some fresh veggies and whole grain pasta to mix into your hamburger meat. Little Sis compared whole grain vs. white pasta on our blog and that is available in the expansion section.

When you are spending that food budget, how much food is in your food? There are plenty of websites that will give you nutritional information about real foods such as: Self Nutrition Data, http://nutritiondata.self.com/

B) Cost per week or month: How much are you REALLY spending on food?

Before you decide you can't afford healthier food, understand where you are spending your food dollars.

Baby Step Action: Write down all the money you spend on food and beverages for 2 weeks and where you spend it. This is not to make you feel bad or to say that you should never buy anything at the ball park again, but when you are unaware of where you are spending your money on food then you are not in charge of HOW you spend your money on food. Unaccounted for food expenditures mean that your grocery bill is not an accurate reflection of your food costs and that you are not in the driver's seat for making actual choices about what you can and can't afford, and what you want to eat.

Not a budgeter? Many people do budget for food, but if you don't (or are willing to admit that you don't stick to it), that's okay, you can still play and win this game! Collect credit card information or receipts for the last month or two that will give you an average that you are actually spending at grocery stores / farmer's markets, and everywhere else per week. If you don't have this information, save it or write it down for the next few weeks to see what you are spending.

Now consider how much you would have to spend at the grocery store / farmer's market if you took ¾'s or ½ of what you are spending in 'other places' and added it to what you normally spend at the grocery store. A few more planned snacks or travel mugs of coffee, tea or water might knock down that expense barrier between you and real food.

C) Considering cost of healthcare / ill health:

Take a risk assessment or two such as those provided by:
The American Diabetes Association: http://www.diabetes.org/are-you-at-risk/diabetes-risk-test/
The American Heart Association:
http://www.heart.org/HEARTORG/Conditions/More/ToolsForYourHeartHealth/Heart-Health-Risk-Assessments-from-the-American-Heart-Association_UCM_306929_Article.jsp
or The American Cancer Society :
http://www.cancer.org/healthy/toolsandcalculators/index

A risk assessment may help you determine how urgent is the need to budget with long term health in mind. Preventing (or lessening the chances of) diabetes, cancer and heart disease is an investment with financial, physical and emotional payoffs!

And finally – I know, this is a busy chapter, but truly your current and long term health is the driving force for making better food choices - now that you have all of this information and realize that not every dollar spent on food is equal in terms of nutrition or health consequences, HOW do you cut back on those expenditures at 'other food places' thereby expanding the amount of money available to spend on real food?
In order to cut down the 'Other Food Place (OFP)' spending the Sis sisters:
• take lunch to work and/or school,
• pack snacks or meals for outings,
• keep snacks in the car for emergencies,

- make coffee or tea at home in the morning and pack it for trips,
- take re-fillable water bottles with us wherever we go, and
- keep ingredients in the pantry and/or freezer that can make a very quick meal.

We sound pretty obnoxious, don't we? Admittedly, this is our ideal list and just like everyone else, we sometimes end up spending money on food in unintended places, but it is a lot less frequent and these actions can return a lot of money to the real food budget.

Your final Baby Step in Chapter 11 is to pick one or more of the above methods for cutting back on 'other food place' spending and commit to a period of time you will execute that real food saving method. You can do it!

Details and links on how we (usually) avoid the 'OFPs' can be found in the expansion section.

Wrapping Up the Action: Baby Steps for Baby Step #11: You Can Afford Health Food

11-1) Compare nutrition labels for some processed item you buy with the ingredients for something made from scratch. This can be challenging, but well worth the time. Alternatively, search the label of your processed food for fruits, vegetables, and fiber. These are often the first things to go during processing. Also take note of the amount of sugar and salt in that little package.

11-2) Follow the steps above to figure out what you are REALLY spending on food.

11-3) Take a risk assessment or two to better understand your risk for developing a preventable disease such as Type II diabetes, heart disease or some cancers.

11-4) Commit to stopping one or more practices of buying food at places other than the grocery store / farmer's market. Make sure you plan on a way to replace the previous method, such as making coffee at home or keeping snack packs (plastic containers or bags of cereal, dried fruit, nuts or granola bars, apples, etc.) in the car.

(Available in Workbook)

INSPIRATION:

Many organizations tout the health benefits of weight loss. The National Heart, Lung and Blood Institute (NIH, 2014) states that the advantages of weight loss are lowering blood pressure, fats in the blood, and blood sugar.[47] The American Diabetes Association recommends that you "stay at a healthy weight, eat well and be active" (ADA, 2014)[48] to reduce your risk of diabetes. One of the easiest ways to lose weight is

Baby Steps to Better Health / Baby Step #11   93.

to increase your intake of vegetables and fruit over other choices. Remember Pre-emptive Produce? Besides taking up space in your belly, vegetables and fruits are very, very good for you from a nutritional standpoint. US News & World Report shared a Harvard study in which a plant-strong diet (one which included modest amounts of fish and lean meat with an emphasis on veggies) lowered blood pressure and therefore chances of developing cardiovascular disease by as much as 30%.[49] The same study also showed improvements in weight control, skin and digestive health. There is inspiration for everyone in a healthy diet!

EXPANSION:

I) Expansion on having and using leftovers to save money
II) Planning to avoid Other Food Places
III) Cheap Recipes!

I) Having and using leftovers.

Where would I be without leftovers? I can answer that. I'd be standing in line in the hospital cafeteria waiting to pay too much for food that is not very good or very healthy. So I bring leftovers to work. Now I know some of you are thinking, "What leftovers? My family eats almost all of whatever I cook! There are no leftovers!" Clearly you are not plagued by an inadequacy complex that compels you to prepare enough food for the hordes that might drop in without warning. And I'm glad if you are not saddled with that particular compulsion as this leaves you able to use your own free will and CHOOSE to make more food. More food = more leftovers.

Now, I am not relegating you to eating dry meatloaf every night for 3 days because you made extra. Honest! Some dishes are nice leftover, or frozen a week later but you can also make extra of the components of a meal and you can mix and match to create new and exciting (for lunch) meals jiffy quick.

I always intentionally make too much of the following:
brown rice,
quinoa,
sautéed vegetables,
cous cous,
sautéed greens,
noodles or pasta,
sauces or dressings,
roasted vegetables,
meat (when we have it – getting rare lately!),
and even nut butter sandwiches.

Baby Steps to Better Health / Baby Step #11

Having all of these leftovers around provides you with the building blocks you need to make meals that do not 'feel' like eating boring old leftovers. (They also provide you with the luxurious ability to create quick dinners with half the work already done.)

Whenever you sauté vegetables, whenever you BUY vegetables, especially when they are on sale, don't think about one meal. Think about several meals.

Take the following sautés all prepared in the oil of your choice:

Zucchini, Eggplant and Spinach with Garlic, Onion and Italian spices
• Allocate some for making pasta sauce by adding diced or crushed tomatoes;
• Allocate some to the freezer for another night's pasta sauce; and
• Allocate some to the refrigerator all by it's lonesome to add to rice, quinoa, pita bread or over salad for lunch.

Peppers (any color or all colors), Green Beans and Onions with Salt and Pepper
• Allocate some to serve with tempeh or meat that night;
• Allocate some to the fridge for making an omelette; and
• Allocate some to the refrigerator for the same punitive treatment received by the poor zucchini, i.e. leftovers for lunchtime (when mixed with grain, wrap, pita or salad).

Leeks, Cabbage, Salt, Pepper and Marjoram (go light on the marjoram – a little goes a long way)
• Allocate some to serve as a side dish for dinner;
• Allocate some to the freezer to use in a casserole or bean dish; and
• Of course, relegate some to the lunchtime penal colony on the bottom shelf of the fridge.

Peppers, Tomatoes, Sun-dried Tomatoes and Onions with Cumin and Chili pepper
• Allocate some as the basis for your chili – be it with veggies, meat or a plant-based product;
• Freeze some for chili or enchiladas another night; and
• Place some in the lunchtime section awaiting mixage with frozen corn or rice or tortilla chips.

How much of each spice? Is that what you are wondering just about now? Well of course it depends on how much you are making, but start low and go slow is the mantra for starting to do your own seasoning. Taste as you go and add more. Be especially gentle with salt, garlic, soy sauce and hot things as they can easily be overdone.

Baby Steps to Better Health / Baby Step #11					95.

II) Planning to Avoid Other Food Places (OFPs)

How did people pack lunches before Ziploc containers, thermoses and Sponge Bob lunchboxes? A tin pail with a sweet potato, that's how. Wow, that was a long time ago, and no I am not that old and was never sent to school like that.

Organization is a key component to avoiding spending money in 'OFP's'. Here is a plan that works for us.

As discussed in the expansion section of chapter 9 we plan 1 – 2 weeks of meals, including lunches and shopping in advance. For a refresher on this see the expansion section in chapter 9.

Another key component in avoiding OFPs is little plastic containers. Goodness knows I don't want to add more plastic to the environment, but at least they are re-usable, right? Besides the routine of packing servings of fruit, veggie and snack mixes in cups to be selected for lunch, we also use these to take with us on outings or errands as a snack. Snacking is a prime source of OFP use. I often find that if I offer a snack cup of trail mix, or an apple both my child and I can discover whether or not we are actually hungry or we are just coveting the doughnut available at the gas station convenience store. I'm not going to condemn you for buying a doughnut once in a while but, again, knowing where our food dollars are going helps us make better choices. Likewise, knowing whether we are craving a sweet distraction or reward or are actually hungry is a valuable lesson in distinction and control….for both us and our children. So pack those little cups with healthier (and cheaper when purchased in bulk) crackers, cereal, dried fruits and nuts, fruits and veggies and be ready when the OFPs are beckoning.

An adjunct to the law of little plastic container packing is the 'pack as you put away' law. When cleaning up dinner, go ahead and put the leftovers in a couple of containers that can go straight in a lunchbox for school or work. I have access to a microwave at work, so my leftover portion goes right into a glass dish with a lid. For school, where there is no microwave, we sometimes put some in a glass container to microwave in the am before putting in a thermos, or just scoop some out in the morning, but it sure saves time to pack as you put away. In addition, when you are chopping a veggie that someone in the house likes raw, chop a little extra and put it in a little plastic container…. Yes, you are going to need to acquire some little plastic containers.

III) Cheap Recipes

Naturally Sweet Sweet Potatoes(p217)
Leftover Mashed Potato Leek Soup(p231)
Shweet Potato Stew(p234)
Cold Kickin' Soup(p228) (great to help beat a cold)
Lentil, Mushroom and Sweet Potato Soup(p232)

Slow Cooker Vegetable, Bean and Barley Stew(p236)
Slow Cooker Creamy Tomato Soup(p235)
Slow Cooker Creamed Lentil Soup(p230)
Belly Warming American Black Bean Soup(p227)
Chickpea Salad Sammies(p165)
Slow and Simple Tortillas, Beans and Rice(p192)
Pakistani Lentil Kima(p182)
Power Tabbouleh(p186)
Chipotle Roasted Sweet Potatoes(p166)
Leftoverlicious Lentil Casserole(p174)
30 Minute Bean and Bulgur Chili(p162)
Baja Hummus (p121) (Hummus is much cheaper homemade and nutritionally dense!)
Garbanzorange Hummus(p123)
Navy Bean Herb Hummus(p124)
Lemony Roast Garlic Hummus(p123)
Nutty Lunch Dip(p125)

CHAPTER 12: Baby Step 12 – A Grocery Store Strategy That Feeds Your Healthy Food Habit

INFORMATION: There are barriers to buying real food in the grocery store.

Some of the barriers to buying real food are external, which is to say that they arise because of the way that food is sold. Some of those barriers are internal, which is to say that we raise them ourselves, by our choices and our habits. Like so many of our normal self-maintenance routines, food shopping is very much an act of habit. If you have not been in the habit of seeking out and buying healthier food, it becomes awfully easy to miss in the market. And if your market is set up like most markets, they're not making it any easier for you to get to those real food goodies. We'd like to offer some specific actions and strategies you can take to the market with you so you come out with a healthier haul. These actions are based on three critical facts about food and grocery stores. 1) Most real food spoils. 2) Much of the food sold in the average grocery store does not spoil. 3) The grocery store is a for-profit business, not a purveyor of health.

1) Most Real Food Spoils

Regardless of whatever your individual food orientation (vegetarian, meat & potatoes lover, fruitarian, pescatarian), many of the healthiest choices you can make, many of the real foods that will provide your bod with optimum nutrition, spoil. They turn grotty. They become sludge or compost depending on what you eat. Some folks believe that the earlier you get these bits into your body – the fresher they are, the more good they will do you.

Let me couch this by saying that there are some perfectly legitimate real food items that take so long to spoil that we could fairly say that they basically don't spoil. I would here be referring to things like dried beans, grains, nuts, some fats, vinegars, and dried fruits and veggies. You get my drift here. These are live food items that have been lightly processed to bring them into a more shelf stable form. They have not had much, if anything, added to them.

The truth is, if you add together the food that *will* spoil and the slightly altered but still real food dried beans and fruits etc, they still make up a pretty low percentage of what's available to you at the grocery store for eating. Let's consider the areas of the store where these real food gems live. I'm not telling you anything revolutionary here – lots of fantastic bloggers and writers have clued us in to the trick of the grocery store: the perimeter. What's on the perimeter? The fridges. If your store has the cold part somewhere else – just replace the word perimeter with that location. You want to go to the cold place because you want to buy a lot of your groceries in the area with the food that spoils.

As supermarkets expand their offerings and their services there are many more ways to entice the average shopper to impulse buy on their way to real food. My neighborhood Wegman's has a bakery and a prepared foods section that boasts a seating area with a kid zone and a fireplace. It's really nice – no lie, but it doesn't necessarily help me stick to my menu and shopping plan. To combat the bounty of wonder that is the modern grocery store, I basically walk the same path through the store every time and only deviate to pick up a particular item – and then return to my regular path. If I didn't put it on the list I don't need it, and if I don't need it, there's no reason for me to walk through an aisle of culinary genius or marketing insanity to get it.

Spoiler alert for the ACTION section… Next time you go to the market, notice your strategy.

2) Much of the Food in the Store Does Not Spoil

There is a giant category of food at the grocery store that never spoils because it, quite frankly, has a lot of crap added to it to ensure that it can sit indefinitely on that grocery shelf until it hits the magic sale price, or the coupon comes out in the Sunday flier, or whatever, and then those goods get transferred from the grocery store shelf to the pantry where they also sit indefinitely. In order to make it possible for these foods to sit on the shelf, producers often add chemicals, known as preservatives, to ensure shelf life. Many preservatives are sodium based and as a result, many shelf stable products are extremely high in salts. While there are sometimes additives in perishable foods, they are much less common, and much less necessary.

There are lists all over the internet of food additives and preservatives that aren't good for you. Here at the pantry we recommend resources at the Center for Science in the Public Interest. They provide a list of additives that you can read about, and they have them broken down into categories of relative safety and harm or potential harm. I would challenge you some day to take the part of the list of additives that CPSI suggests we all avoid and look at it while you're in an aisle at the store – one of those interior aisles with box after box of quick easy dinner time fixes. You're going to find the ingredients from that list. You're going to find them everywhere. You're going to find them in the foods you never thought you'd have to question. You'll also find them in the blue microwave popcorn – c'mon you knew that was a bad idea. You're going to find them in the foods that they're marketing to your children. You're going to find them in many, many grocery items that don't spoil. So you don't have to believe that a food must be alive in order to think that perishable food is better for you – you just have to believe that avoiding harmful chemicals is a good idea.

Spoiler alert for the ACTION section: While you're learning about all this stuff, carry a list of harmful additives when you go to the market.

3) The Grocery Store is a For Profit Business

I know you know this, but I think sometimes we forget that grocery stores are businesses like so many others. They exist to sell you food, and it is in their best interest for you to buy those foods at the highest price possible, and to need to come to the store often, to cultivate your loyalty, and to encourage careless and thoughtless shopping so you get a lot and still forget some items from your list. What? That sounds so mean, so awful, so dastardly… Look, I'm not saying every person in your favorite market is trying to pick pocket you. I AM saying that retailers of all kinds do serious research to figure out exactly how to get you to spend as much as possible while in their store. This is not the same goal as helping you get the biggest bang for your buck or improve your diet. This means that their deals are intended largely to bring in new customers and that, for the most part, everyday prices on items that you want to eat are far more important than big sales. I'm not suggesting you ignore sale prices, but pay attention to what you get charged for the food that you WANT to eat more of. Keep an eye on those everyday prices on healthful perishable items.

Spoiler alert for the ACTION section: If you're committed to a particular market, consider the reason for your loyalty.

REFLECTION:

I'm at the grocery store. I've brought the twins (something I try very hard to avoid). One of them is chasing me with a package of purple glitter nail polish and the other is asking in his most polite voice if he can just SHOW me something he saw a few aisles ago; he won't ask me to buy it, he promises. I am maxed out. I have a list but I can't freaking find it. My cell phone is vibrating into my side and I can see from the screen that it's an old friend I've been exchanging voice mail with for months. Calgon take me away indeed. This IS shopping, though. Purchasing the stuff of life happens on regular days with all of their regular promise and regular pitfalls. Despite the purple glitter nail polish pleading (or whatever drives you nuts at the store), we all make it home with some food. Well, at least mostly.

> *12a) Do I find grocery the store stressful? If so, why?*
>
> *12b) Do I shop with a list? Do I stick to the list?*
>
> *12c) How much time do I spend in the produce aisle?*
>
> *(Available in Workbook)*

ACTION: *A Grocery Store Strategy That Feeds Your Healthy Food Habit*

So can all of our eating pitfalls be addressed at the grocery store? No, but a whole lot of them can. If you are eating junk and that junk is available to you in your home, finding a new way to shop would take you a good way down the road to better health. So here we offer the actions we recommend in rehabbing that grocery store strategy.

Action 1) Notice your strategy at the market so you can create a plan for shopping:

• Do you go down every aisle?

• Do you stick to a list or do you let the store dictate what you'll be buying?

• Note how much time you spend in the cold parts of the store.

Step: Create a physical plan for navigating your market to find and buy the real food.

If you are feeling bold you might delineate a section or aisle of the grocery store as off limits. There are aisles in my store to which I only went in researching this book. It was kind of interesting to realize that I'd not been in that aisle and had no idea just how many versions of macaroni and cheese and hamburger helper type 'foods' exist.

Some stores actually have store maps available on line so you can figure out where you really need to be without any of the carefully researched distractions in the market. Take a minute to see if your store's layout is made available to you somewhere that doesn't have an end cap with blue microwave popcorn on it.

Action 2) Carry a list of harmful additives when you go to the market and read your labels.

• Choose 5 non-perishable food items that you customarily buy and check out their ingredients to see what harmful additives they contain.

• Choose 1 (or more) of those that contain harmful ingredients and swap that item out in favor of a real food alternative.

See Baby Step 1 for a reminder of what swapping out is all about.

Action 3) Evaluate your choice of market - Think about why you shop where you shop.

• Is it because they offer amazing deals?

• Is it because they have a great bakery?

- Take note of the everyday prices of perishable foods and make sure you're getting as good a deal as you think. A good food deal is only a good deal if it includes something that actually feeds your body.

Action 4) Work on your shopping list.

Finally and firstly, in order to buy real food at the grocery store, you may well need to start by working on your list. If your list is full of junk food, guess what's going to come home? Secondly, stick to that list. The people who know me well are now flat out laughing at me. I'm not good at sticking to the list – but here's the thing I AM good at sticking to - my path. This is to say that when I stray off list at my local Wegman's, I am most likely in the produce section, the refrigerated natural foods section (where I get organic milk and eggs and crazy healthy bread), or at the olive bar. If you have something bad to tell me about the olive bar, I'd just as soon you kept it to yourself, thank you very much. So make that list and don't go into other parts of the store. You don't need that crap. You really don't. Drift toward the perimeter. Bring a sweater if you must. Real food wants cold. Real food spoils. Real food wants to be eaten sooner rather than later.

Wrapping Up the Action: Baby Steps for Baby Step #12: A Grocery Store Strategy That Feeds Your Healthy Food Habit

12-1) Notice your strategy at the market so you can create a plan for shopping and then create a physical plan for navigating your market to find and buy the real food.

12-2) Carry a list of harmful additives when you go to the market and read your labels.

12-3) Evaluate your choice of market. Think about why you shop where you shop.

12-4) Work on your shopping list.

(Available in Workbook)

INSPIRATION:

Many people get annoyed by the advertisements aimed at young children. We are all familiar with the ads that cause your children to hound you for a certain brand of cereal, shoes, toys or whatever! Many of us explain to our children that most of those items are not as wonderful as the advertisers would like us to believe. What about the grown ups? What about those ads aimed at you? They are all over the grocery store. Remember that advertisers lie. It is their job to stretch the truth. Okay they would probably call it 'spinning' or 'emphasizing added value,' or bringing a product to the attention of an appropriate market rather than lying. When our kids "spin" about their involvement in using blue Silly Putty on the white carpet, we call it lying. Remember

Baby Steps to Better Health / Baby Step #12

that you are being lied to so that someone can make more money. I get a bit angry about the lying for profit and it actually helps me have no desire to put more money in the pockets of those who stretch the truth at the expense of *everyone's* health.

EXPANSION:

You may feel that we ourselves are advertising a bill of goods in regards to the dangers of processed food. We suggest that you do a little of your own research. There are many fine books and documentaries out there to educate and entertain. Both of used books and documentaries for our own learning and growth and found them to be very useful in sharing information with reluctant spouses. Really, nobody wants to hear that their favorite treat is dangerous. It takes some repetition and some different voices to reach a point of decision on changing dietary habits. Those different voices are readily available.

CHAPTER 13: Baby Step #13: Saving on Produce: Shop Smart/Use Smart

INFORMATION: Strategic Shopping Can Save Money

Now that we've recognized all of the ways we spend money on food that may not be the best choice, we'd like to focus on saving money on some of the healthiest food around: produce. Saving on produce tends to fall into two basic categories: 1) spending less and 2) using more (or wasting less if you're into complete grammatical parallels). Both approaches are obviously valid, but the greatest savings (and satisfaction if you're a cheap freak like me) comes from employing methods from both categories to maximize the nutrish for the dinero, moolah, green, whatev. Shopping is more than walking down the aisles getting lured into 'what's for dinner' by the most brightly colored package – it can be a strategic adventure that yields healthy food on a budget! Doesn't that sound exciting?

REFLECTION:

13a) Can you think of some fruits or vegetables that you only eat at certain times of the year?

13b) Do you have any positive associations for those items? (For example, eating cherries on the 4th of July.)

13c) Do you ever try new fruits or veggies because they are on sale?

Click here for workbook / app

Healthy food, which for most folks means adding more produce, is affordable because it satisfies you and prevents spending money on chronic illness. Healthy food is more affordable if you get good at finding it cheap and using it all.

Some of our suggestions for saving money on produce are obvious, but if you're anything like me you tend to get real good about focusing on one strategy and then forget some of the others. Let's run through the possibilities.

ACTION: Saving on Produce: Shop Smart/Use Smart

Saving on the Front End: Shop Smart

1) Shop Seasonally: Ever notice that tomatoes get cheaper when it's blazing hot in your region? That grapefruit gets wicked inexpensive in winter? This is all about season. So many of us have forgotten about shopping seasonally because thanks to international exports, breeding for durability, and masterful storage by food producers, we have grown accustomed to getting just about anything we want any time of year. When you take advantage of sales in season you are far more likely getting the freshest (and most delicious) produce you can buy at a good price. It's all about good nutrish for less dish. Sure a tomato is a delicious addition to a sandwich, salad or open mouth, but not so much when it is mealy and flavorless. You might consider trying something new, cheaper and more tasty than an off-season tomato while you wait for the good stuff.

2) Double that Load: When the price is really good, get a lot and just eat it like it's going out of style. Eat salad every meal in Spring. Eat it until you can't bear the sight of that super fresh super nutritious bright green snap pea. Know why that's okay? Because if you're shopping in season, right about the time you burn out, it will be time for the next wave. Taking advantage of sale prices by buying a lot also allows you to save for later times - which we'll discuss in more detail later.

3) Find that Farmer: I know, I know you've heard it before and if you aren't into farmer's markets you don't likely want to hear it again, but the truth is that farm markets are often the best place to get the freshest high quality produce at the best price. They also allow you to try your hand at a little wheeling and dealing. In years when the squirrels take too many of my 'maters, we negotiate with one of our favorite local guys for big boxes of tomatoes so that I can save some. Make relationships. These folks will share amazing produce AND knowledge and if you're smart you'll ask enough questions that you can…

4) Grow Some: Okay, okay you're not a gardener. I get it. Truth is most folks can save at least a little dough, or at least improve their ingredients, by planting a couple of pots of herbs. There are plenty of veggies and fruits that can be done small-scale and if you have more room, it might be wise to consider which veggies you eat the most of and which cost you the most at the store in order to maximize your savings with your efforts in the dirt.

5) Shop/Grow Cooperatively: If you garden and so does your pal, make some deals so you can make the most of your space but still enjoy a variety of veggies. If you don't garden, work with a friend so you can help each other by taking advantage of sales for one another. If you text, this is REALLY easy. It goes something like this: Me: "At Weggie's, Org Strawberries 3.50/lb. Want some?" Shopping Pal: "YES!! Get 3!" There, it's that simple.

Saving on the Back End….er, Other End: Use More/Waste Less

1) Freeze those Bits: Got more beans than you can handle? Strawberries starting to look dusky before you've used them? Peas or broccoli coming in from the garden in quantities too small to use at one shot? Experiment with small batch freezing. I've been doing this all summer with berries, peas, broccoli florets and greens. I have a tray set in the freezer with wax paper for berries and a simple sheet of wax paper for the veggies. I wash, trim (if needed), lay them on the wax paper, check the next day and put them into a storage bag. Done. Slowly gathering quantities for the winter, just like those pesky squirrels who eat my tomatoes… This should probably generate some compassion for them from me… Hmmmm…

2) Be Aware: More often than not when produce goes bad in my fridge it's because I forgot it was there. Something got shoved on top of something else and something got shoved to the back and the container opened and now there's this weird smell… yeah. You've been there. I've been trying to be a lot more aware of what's in there by at least once a day (while I'm getting stuff, not like an extra trip) taking a peek through both of those bins and eyeballing the fridge generally (I often have too much produce for just the bins). I've also adopted the practice when I get home from the market of pulling things out of the bins and consolidating BEFORE I add the new bits. Now I know exactly what's in there. When you know what's in there, there's a better chance you will use it especially if you…

3) Develop an Early Warning System: When you know you've had some produce too long, move it somewhere obvious. I've seen folks do this a variety of ways – a special bin in the fridge for things that must be used pronto, a list of items to use up ASAP, a quick change of the menu or lunch leftovers to accommodate those fragile veggies. I tend to pull them out of the crisper for easy viewing and adapt my menus to take advantage of them. Make it easy on yourself; adopt a system of some kind. I can't speak for you, but if I rely on my head to do all of this, I'll have a fridge full of yuck and P.U.

4) Try Some Canning or Drying: I have both canned and dried produce, and to be honest I'm not in love with either process, but I will can some tomatoes and I will dry me some herbs. I find the payoff on both of these to be well worth the effort. If I have enough berries I will also do some syrup or jam, but I usually just stuff those directly into my giant gaping maw.

5) Alter the Food Format to Buy Some Time: Got bananas that are past their prime? You know what I'm going to say, right? Banana bread is yesterday's answer (although it's always a good one). Super soft bananas are great for baking LOTS of healthy bits like cookies, pancakes, just about anything that you usually put fat into and that is meant to be enjoyed sweet. You can also, of course, peel and freeze them for non-dairy smoothies and ice cream. For savory produce savings, see if you can turn your veggies into a slaw or fresh pickle in order to buy some time. Vinegar is magical and will give you some more time to enjoy those bits. Delish, frugal, and oh so satisfying.

Wrapping up the Action: Baby Steps for Baby Step #13: Saving on Produce: Shop Smart/Use Smart

13-1) Notice (or ask) if your grocery store makes the origin of produce available. Some stores place signs to show what is locally grown.

13-2) Notice (or ask) if your store has a reduced section or cart for produce that has seen better days. Take it home and cook it/ slice it / eat it right away.

13-3) Make note of which items you buy seasonally and which you buy year round. Try making a switch and see if you can taste the difference or appreciate the price drop.

13-4) Decide which you would like to try first – freezing, planting your own, drying or canning. Learn something about it and give it a go!

13-5) Get to know the people who work in the produce section at your grocery store – they might see you and say, "Hey I was just about to add some red peppers to the markdown area, you want some?"

13-6) Find out if there are any farmer's markets or any farms that provide shares of community supported agriculture (CSA)[50] in your neck of the woods.

13-7) Develop an early warning system for food that needs to be eaten ASAP.

(Available in Workbook)

INSPIRATION:

Remind yourself why you wish to eat more healthfully.

"At lunch you order steamed vegetables because you're remembering that you have a heart too. You feel humbled by your heart, it works so hard. You want to thank it. You give your heart a little pat." — Aimee Bender, The Girl in the Flammable Skirt

"Give me juicy autumnal fruit, ripe and red from the orchard."
From "Give Me the Splendid Silent Sun" — Walt Whitman[51]

EXPANSION:

This expansion section is a love song to kale. Not literally, but kale, like many other vegetables is one of those that many people quickly profess to hating, or avoiding or never trying but being quite sure that the results would be disastrous should they place some kale in their mouth. But besides being a powerhouse for nutrition, it is also available in big bags or big bundles, lasts fairly well and can be prepared many ways. Even Little Sis thought she didn't like it! Here is her journey from kale dubious to kale

Baby Steps to Better Health / Baby Step #13

enthusiast. It is a lesson for letting a vegetable grow on you, complete with lots of recipes. (Sorry about the 'grow on you.')

Buuuuut, you're saying "I don't like kale. I mean I've never liked kale. Okay, I've never had kale, but I don't like spinach and that's kind of like kale, so why should I eat kale? Surely there's something else I could eat – how about just something else green? Because I'm pretty sure I don't like kale…" Or something. No, I'm not mocking you. I'm giving you the speech from the monkeys in my head when Bigg Sis suggested I eat kale. How about instead of eating a whole lot of something else that's okay but not nearly as good for you, you just try some kale? There's a LOT of ways to go about this, so I'm going to help you out. I'm going to just lay out a bunch of kale goodness on a kind of sliding scale of how much you need to like kale – kay? I'll start with the doubters.

Step 1: Surely you know what's coming. It could only be a slightly frozen fruity concoction into which you camouflage some kale. Who's to be the wiser? Know who drinks kale smoothies? My 6 year olds. With delight. Yup, all that leafy green goodness just slides right on in them. There are a TON of kale smoothie recipes out there. We've got a few in the smoothie section(p224).

Step 2: I can't speak for anybody else, but creamed spinach changed my whole relationship with greens. I had avoided them religiously before I tried creamed spinach, and then I was in like Flynn (who's Flynn anyway, and what is he in?). Bigg Sis and I avoid dairy these days, but that doesn't mean we can't have some creamy stuff, and her Creamed Kale(p212) takes me right back to that creamed spinach love.

Step 3: Soup is a great way to ease your way into all kinds of food. Whatever you're not sure about is dancing around in a bowl with all kinds of bits you actually DO want to eat. Putting kale in soup bumps up that nutrition hugely, adds some texture and color and makes for a fine and dandy meal. I recently made White Bean and Kale Stew from Kathy Hester's *The Vegan Slow Cooker*. Fan-flipping tastic. Ever put balsamic vinegar in soup? I have now, and you should too. Fix it and forget it fo' sho'.

Step 4: Maybe you've come to believe that you might actually like kale. Time to try some Wilted Greens. Tear the leaves from the stems of a whole bunch of kale. Warm some olive oil in a pan, add some crushed garlic. Add the kale and cook it until it is intensely green and softer, stirring occasionally. Sprinkle with salt. Add raisins and toasted pine nuts if you're feeling fancy. Delish.

Step 5: Raw and Massaged… No you haven't just flipped over to the kind of book you don't want to read in public. I'm talking massaged kale. Yes, I'm serious. Try Ani Phyo's Kale, Avocado and Sprouts Salad. It is absolutely straight up fantastic. The avocado works to dress the kale. So fresh, so yummy.

Step 6: Kale as Salad. Tonight I needed to slap something super nutritious together for myself in a jiff. So I grabbed the bunch of kale I bought this morning (my plants are recovering from a massive harvest a few weeks ago) and tore off enough to create a big old bed in the bottom of a pasta bowl, cut up about a quarter of an avocado, added about 2/3 c of leftover slow cooker barley, black bean and corn burrito(p161) filling, topped with a spoonful of sunflower cheese(p121) and sprinkled on a little red wine vinegar and some salt. Fast and superb.

Give kale and any other vegetable you haven't tried a chance. Especially when it's in season and on sale. There is nothing like being nourished for the long term with reasonably priced food. Real food.

CHAPTER 14: Baby Step #14: Nourishment Beyond Food

INFORMATION: Nourishment is about more than food.

Merriam Webster's on-line dictionary defines nourishment as food or nutriment[52]. Nutriment is defined as "something that nourishes or promotes growth, provides energy, repairs body tissues and maintains life[53]." The popularity of books like "Chicken Soup for the Soul" affirms the notion that we seek nourishment for mind, body and spirit. It takes more than food to cover all of those bases.

REFLECTION:

I believe that part of the battle for creating a healthy lifestyle is identifying what nourishes you. Taste buds are not the only players in the satisfaction game. A nourishing meal or experience is satisfying because you have been nourished, i.e., your body, mind or spirit has been strengthened, guided, fed, nurtured, sustained, encouraged, cultivated, supported, fostered, developed and/or promoted. I'd like to see a McDonald's french fry do that all by itself. Mind you, a McDonald's french fry eaten with friends….. or after basketball practice….. or on a date…… or any other physically, emotionally or spiritually fulfilling activity is another story. So, it's not always the french fry that satisfied you, but the company or the circumstances in which you ate that fry.

> *14a) What makes you feel good for a prolonged period of time? What do you talk or think about a day, a week, or a year later?*
>
> *14b) Why do you find unhealthy food (pick your fave) satisfying? Is it the convenience? Is it buying something? Is it the restaurant atmosphere or sneaking something once the kids have gone to bed? Is it the taste, the texture? Is it having someone make something for you? Does it represent a break from an activity that you find difficult or draining?*
>
> *14c) Do you plan nourishing activities to feed yourself and possibly your family in body, mind and spirit?*
>
> *(Available in Workbook)*

To add some nourishment, you have to figure out what nourishes you. If you can recognize some truths about what nourishes you, it might be easier to get more nourishment and less 'processed food Ka-Pow sugar/fat and salt taste' into your life.

ACTION: Nourish Yourself: Nourishment Beyond Food

1) Check your self-worth.

In order to add some nourishment, you must believe that you are worth nourishing. It is easier to believe that you are worth nourishing when you are well nourished. "Them that's got, shall get," right? Kind of twisted, but I believe it's true. Sometimes you have to act like you are there before you've actually arrived. You have to decide and act as though you are worth nourishing even if you don't believe it. This approach is like smiling at yourself in the mirror when you don't feel very up. It makes you feel better. Steve Martin says you can't play a sad song on the banjo. It's also hard to be sad when you are smiling. It's also easier to choose healthy food once you have experienced nourishment. But you have to pay attention. You can't attribute feelings, behavior and choices to feelings, behavior and choices, unless you are paying attention.

So again, ask yourself:

> *14d) Why do I choose what I choose?*
>
> *14e) Am I trying to nourish myself? – remember all of those wonderful meanings of nourished: strengthened, guided, fed, nurtured, sustained, encouraged, cultivated, supported, fostered, developed and/or promoted.*
>
> *14f) What nourishes me?*
>
> *14g) How do I get more of what nourishes me in my life?*

Pay attention to what nourishes you.

2) Experiment with Conscious Choices

Consciousness about your choices may make you aware of more choices, both food and non-food, available to you. If they are nourishing choices, you may ultimately find them to be more satisfying than what you currently choose. I often use Lent as a time to remind myself of what a certain indulgence means in my life. When I give it up, I either miss it terribly or find that it was not so important to me after all. That is how I was able to reduce my sugar intake. I found that after 40 days of nothing sweet I found most sweets unappetizingly sweet and by the end I didn't miss them as much as I thought I would. Giving up fiction did not have the same result. I missed it very much and appreciated it more when I returned to it. In fact, I think I chose my books more carefully because I wanted to read really good books. Since those days of Lenten deprivation I have found it very helpful to ADD something for Lent – some devotional practice or amount of quiet time or time spent to help others and I find that to be very nourishing. What could you give up or add to your life to challenge your conscious decision-making?

Baby Step #14 is really a life-long journey, but even long journeys can be taken in baby steps. I certainly have made steps forward and backwards in learning what, and then pursuing what nourishes me. While 'Battening down the hatches' in survival mode or giving up things entirely can give us clarity about what we actually require to survive, finding and pursuing what nourishes us in body, mind and spirit can help us survive and grow with grace, and with respect for ourselves and for others. It's not easy. I have to remind myself that like all of the baby steps, an itty bitty baby step forward in nourishing myself rather than just filling the tank is still a step forward. In fact it nourishes me to attempt, to succeed, to fail, and to try again. I remember and treasure this process long after the memory of tasty treats has faded.

Wrapping Up the Action: Baby Steps for Baby Step #14: Nourishment Beyond Food

14-1) Think about what nourishes you. Perhaps list a few non-food actions/activities or habits that nourish you.

14-2) Pay attention to the choices you are making and be honest with yourself about whether or not they nourish you either physically or spiritually.

14-3) Choose some items or actions of genuine tried and true nourishment and add them to your routine. Note whether or not they have any impact on how you feel.

(Available in Workbook)

EXPANSION:

Bad weather brings out the survivor in us, doesn't it? Threats to our electricity, our ability to drive (with all the inherent loss of access to food and other stuff), ability to do our job, and our plans in general, are indeed very upsetting threats. Some of us bring in the outdoor furniture or delicate plants, some of us check the batteries in the flashlights, some of us buy lots of bread and milk, some of us check the firewood, blankets and maybe even fuel supply for the generator.

It is a giant step in our culture to go from: "You deserve a break today…. Treat yourself…. A moment for you…. You deserve the best…. Because you're worth it," and all the other attempts by advertisers to get us to reward ourselves by purchasing their products to: "Batten down the hatches!" We don't have to batten down very often, do we? Left to our own devices and the influence of Madison Avenue we've become quite accustomed to having our favorite food or at least something we genuinely like when we eat - every time we eat. Why not? Who wouldn't choose what they like over what they dislike? Restaurants, convenience stores, vending machines and the center aisles of the grocery store are all too happy to provide our favorites, with plenty of questionable additives to keep them from spoiling, and to make them easy to prepare.

My fellow nurses and I marvel over the number of patients who will say, "I can't eat that," or "I don't eat that" when offered hospital food, not because of allergies or being vegetarian, or gluten-free, but simply because they don't like it, or it's not what they are used to or it's not prepared the way they usually fix it. Why should the nurses be surprised? Nurses are surprised because nursing is a fast-paced, 'batten down the hatches' kind of job. With far too many tasks to complete in far too little time, we are in survival – and patient survival – mode pretty much all the time. As a result, we just don't always understand that patients who are recovering or depressed or feeling lousy but not in danger, continue to behave within the rules of this culture. "You deserve something that you like, why not your favorite?" And so when the patient complains about the food, we ask them what they want, call the fine people in nutritional services, get the patient's request filled if at all possible, (no matter if it's not terribly healthy), and then make jokes in the nurse's station about how we work in a spa rather than a hospital. (Some of the high cost of American health care, this spa mentality, but we won't go there today).

I am not trying to say these patients' behavior is bad or wrong. It is our culture and it is what it is; these stories from the nurses' station, however, do offer some insight into the difficulty of improving eating habits and trying to maintain a healthy weight in this American culture. How is a person supposed to feel satisfied by a meal or a snack if that meal or snack represents less than what one likes, or is less than what is 'deserved,' or somehow less than what society says is good, best, or one's right?

Sometimes after work when I've been out of the house for 14 hours and running around for about 11 of those, I get home and feel ravenously hungry. If I don't pay attention I will overeat and sometimes choose the least healthy option in the house before realizing that I'm full and not running and my feet hurt less and I can slow down and take care of myself. I just caught myself doing it again last night, so I'm going to pack one last healthy item in my lunch bag to eat on the way home. That will take the edge off of feeling ravenous and allow me to come into the house and nourish myself by sitting down, relaxing and catching up with my husband and son. They nourish me (when I spend time with them!). Allowing myself to be still after a very busy day nourishes me. Reading nourishes me. Making things nourishes me. Meditating or praying nourishes me. So many things other than a quick fix of a Ka-Pow dose of sugar, fat or salt nourish me. And it is lovely when I pay attention and care for myself enough to seek out deep nourishment over shallow satisfaction.

CHAPTER 15: Baby Step 15 – Shake Your Groove Thing: Work Some Activity Into Your Busy Life

INFORMATION: Exercise is important to your health.

According to the American Heart Association, exercise reduces the risk for cardiovascular disease, diabetes, obesity, and hypertension.[54] But it's not just that exercise is good for you; LACK of exercise is bad for you. Lack of physical activity places people at risk for developing high blood pressure, coronary artery disease, anxiety and depression, some cancers, and obesity.[55] Of course you know all of this already, but after the last chapter where we encouraged you to nourish yourself because you are indeed worth nourishing, we thought we'd slip in a reminder that there are actually heavy-duty consequences to health choices.

REFLECTION:

In our baby steps series, we've talked about food. Okay, we've talked a WHOLE LOT about food. We've also talked a great deal about how we think about ourselves and how we think about food, the ways we use food appropriately and inappropriately, the ways our culture portrays and uses food. We've talked about honoring and respecting ourselves enough to nourish ourselves. But we haven't talked about everything we need to do to be in better health. Heck, in some ways we haven't even scratched the surface, but even in the interest of keeping it simple, we're not done. There is an elephant in the room, and I'm not talking about my maternity pictures…

Bigg Sis and I started with food because… we really like food… AND we truly believe that eating more healthfully makes all other aspects of self-care easier. But even with all the healthy food in the world, there's something simple our bodies need that we've not talked about. It's time to get a move on. NONONONONO, don't close the book! Don't leave because this is NOT where I tell you exactly how much to exercise every day and how to use some equation to calibrate that perfectly with what you're eating. Don't leave because this is NOT where I have some miraculous contraption that will give you a great butt. Don't leave because I have no interest in having you look at your body to find fault with it.

Stay here and do a little thinking about how much you move your body. I don't know you – you may run marathons. I know I wanted to. You may have an exercise routine down, and if you DO, that is awesome. If you're like a WHOLE lot of people and you don't have time to have an exercise routine, you hate to exercise, you can't imagine running a marathon being even remotely appealing… stay here and think a little about baby steps.

Baby Steps to Better Health / Baby Step #15

15a) Do any of your leisure activities involve being active?

15b) Is there an activity from your past that you enjoyed? A sport or activity you participated in in school?

15c) What activity(ies) look like fun to you?

15d) Does moderate activity feel good?

(Available in Workbook)

Finding motivation for action is a definite concern for many folks struggling to get active. I'd like to offer a few stories about exercise in my life as a demonstration of the importance of realistic goals when considering starting a new exercise plan.

STORY 1

Mr. Little Sis and I had a really rough couple of years. REALLY rough. I had a miscarriage that nearly killed me. Mr. Little Sis got laid off and then Mr. Little Sis' Mom died. Believe it or not there are more bits of woe from that time, but those are the highlights. I was low, I mean not talking to anyone, not wanting to do anything, not wanting to go to the graduate program I'd worked so hard to get into. One day a friend asked me to go to the park and as our dogs cavorted and tried to start trouble with other dogs we talked honestly about my fragile state. When I revealed the utter lack of motivation that seemed to start every day for me, he asked a simple question. "What if you pretended you didn't have a choice? What if you just decided you HAVE to do these things?" It was an interesting perspective. I was attending my graduate program, but was deeply distracted by not WANTING to go because I was so down.

I took his advice to heart and decided to pretend I didn't have a choice about anything. And one of the first things I decided to do was to start taking a slightly longer walk with my dogs every day. I started parking a little farther out in the student lot and walking in to campus. I went back to my old habit of looking for the worst parking spot at the grocery store and forgetting where all the elevators were on campus. I became the stairs. Each step made me feel more alive, more energized, and more in control of my days in a time when I was clearly not in control of much of anything. I began to run and search out my knee joint tolerance level for pavement pounding, building up a little bit, month by month – slower than even the most judicious trainers would recommend. I was renewed and that sense of renewal, physical and mental, carried me for quite some time, through graduate school and a few years beyond until I found myself carrying twins... There's no jogging or baby stepping around that one.

STORY 2

There was a day at my OB's office when I stepped on the scale and I gasped. The nurse said "Honey, let's have you face the other way for the next couple of weeks. I'll let you know if we're getting into a problem area." Yeah. A problem area. My children were 7 and 6 pounds when they were born – pretty big for twins, and I was so big with them that I required a walking stick to raise myself from my mandated bed rest position to standing (in order to pee, of course). The few pictures my husband was brave enough to take during this period show a tired woman with what looks like a balance ball shoved up her weirdly cut shirt. The children were born, and they took some of that weight with them, but not enough. Bed rest and the relatively lower level of physical activity before that time had left me unmotivated, out of shape, and without a starting line at a time when I was averaging about 3 hours of sleep a night.

I don't know what motivated me – whether it was a friend, something I read, or sheer delusional brilliance, but I ordered a pedometer. There was not a lot I could do in terms of serious exercise with infant twins, but I could walk. Heck, I was already walking a lot – back and forth from bedroom to bedroom, back and forth next to the crib, back and forth in the living room doing the bouncy thing, and up and down the hills of my neighborhood with a stroller. While I don't recommend counting many things, there is a value in knowing what you are currently doing if you are attempting to do MORE of anything. The pedometer let me set new goals, add some steps over time and give myself the room I needed to get back into reasonable shape, feeling more like myself, and again a little more in control of my daily existence at a time when I really wasn't in charge at all.

STORY 3

This story is a little more modern. I was recently subjected to surgery on my big toe joint. Apparently I injured that joint at some point and it's been wonky ever since. That wonkiness led to bone spurs. Ignoring bone spurs while you walk aggressively and occasionally run for exercise is, well, not good. So my rock star orthopedist removed all those nasty spurs and I sat on my posterior all the time for two weeks. For a few more weeks after that I sat on my increasing posterior most of the time. I'm not sure how much of my personality has come through in this book, but let's suffice it to say that sitting still is not my strong suit. The difference with my post-surgical exercise prospects was that I couldn't simply begin to exercise again by measuring the steps I was taking and increasing their number, I had to go WAY back. I had to go to a physical therapist and have him move my toes. Step #1 was moving the toes and not beating myself up too badly about the weight gain during my mandated idle time. After moving the toes for a few weeks, I got to take the cumbersome walking boot off and try walking in regular shoes, short distances with ice to follow. At some point in the progression I became stable enough to have our 85 pound dog join me and take a

REAL walk. As for running, rock star orthopedist is not a fan but allowed that I could try it as one part of a multi-faceted approach to exercise. Great.

Baby Steps and Exercise

The point of sharing these stories is to demonstrate a key principle of our beliefs about better nutrition and better health. You have to start where YOU are. Maybe you're ready to run a 5K, maybe you are ready to walk the dog twice a day, or maybe you need to start by wiggling your toes. Doing someone else's next step will not get you further down YOUR path. Changing habits, lives, and bodies requires time and a bit of 'oh so elusive (especially for me) patience' as well as some honest thought.

As with all of our endeavors, the Sis sisters recommend facing exercise with an honest assessment of what you currently do. This is not the same as asking whether or not you go to the gym. Perhaps you also have a canine friend who requires walking, maybe you go on hikes on the weekend, maybe you are a floor nurse and walk ALL DAY LONG. The next question is whether your current level of exercise has you feeling as fit as you'd like to be. If not, the follow up to the honest assessment is to choose one thing you're going to do to increase your fitness level. Execute that plan for a time and see how you feel. I know, I know you don't have time – seriously I get it. Choose something small that you can add that doesn't make much time. It's much easier to adjust your schedule 15 minutes at a time than to add an hour of activity all at once.

ACTION: Work Some Activity Into Your Busy Life

Baby Steps to Fitness: Some Really Easy Places to Start

Parking Lots – Stop looking for the best space, look for the worst, or as bad as you can tolerate and walk it.

Stairs – Take them all or part of the way to your destination. If you work on the 5th floor and can't possibly walk up five flights of stairs, then walk up one and then take the elevator. Eventually you can walk up 2, then 3, etc.

Public Transit – get off a stop earlier and walk it in.

Don't use a riding mower – unless you have way more land than you can cover. Use a mower you walk behind.

Extra Stairs – when going up or down the stairs at home, repeat the trip for a boost.

A Short Walk – take a few minutes sometime during your day for a short walk – the fresh air and natural light can do wonders for you.

Errand on Foot – If you live where you CAN actually walk to the market or the library, do it. There are all manner of carts and wagons in the world that can help you bring your loot home.

Enlist a Friend – we all have friends who are more fit than we are (Bigg Sis is SUPER scary fit). Observe, listen, pay attention. What do they do that we don't do? Can we borrow some of their habits, activities, or ask them to take a walk?

Try Something New – maybe you didn't like to swim as a kid and haven't done it since – our tastes do change, perhaps the pool is the place for you.

Dance – Put on music that, for you, is undeniably dance material and dance - with your family, with your friends, or all by yourself. This is fun, very cheap, and does not require you to buy any special stuff!

Videos – If you are grooving a little on moving and want to do something a bit organized at home, try an exercise video. Choose one that is at your level, or that offers different levels of ability, and that other people think is fun (assuming you like fun). Make sure you find out how long the workout is, or if it can be broken into pieces so that you can start from YOUR starting point.

Increasing our fitness and activity level doesn't have to mean joining the gym (unless you want it to). What can you do that's a little more than you do today? Where do you park your car at the grocery store? Pick a way to increase your activity level and commit as if you don't have a choice. Like brushing your teeth, activity is something you have to do. As for me, I am making my own toes move again, and I am taking it from there, one healthful step at a time.

Wrapping Up the Action: Baby Steps for Baby Step #15: Work Some Activity Into Your Busy Life

15-1) Consider your current fitness level and honestly assess whether you are where you'd like to be.

15-2) Evaluate your current level of activity. How much are you moving?

15-3) Identify parts of your daily routine where you could reintroduce activity as part of your daily life.

15-4) Try adding one new activity or action to your routine and make note of how you feel as a result.

(Available in Workbook)

EXPANSION:

Just an addition on this theme that is near and dear to my heart… and my blood pressure…and above all, my sanity. There is considerable evidence that exercise improves mental as well as physical health. Not only is there the release of endorphins (pleasure chemicals) that comes with a strong workout, but there is the release of physical and mental stress, a chance to concentrate on what your body is doing instead of what is or isn't happening as you'd like in your life, and a tiredness that helps with relaxing and sleep. Just as we've encouraged you to pay attention to what makes you feel better, what nourishes you, and what healthful foods work for you, pay attention to what kinds of movement work for you and do more of it, or a variation of it…. One step at a time.

As Little Sis mentioned a pedometer was a great starting point for her. There are apps available that will count your steps while carrying your smart phone. Seeing those numbers does make you want to get a few more steps in by walking a little extra or taking the stairs. There are also lots of fitness trackers where you can list goals and record successes. Whatever works to get you moving is a good thing! Now you'll excuse me but I hear some Motown in the background and my groove is indeed shaking – why restrain it?

In Conclusion:

There is no conclusion. Just an on-going journey of learning to savor yourself, learning to savor food that is nourishing and restorative, and learning to hold the line against the influx of messages telling you that cheap and 'easy' is good enough… at least most of the time! Go back to any baby step at any time and just keep stepping the bad out and the good in. Review your steps as needed. Remember that the baby steps still are progress and if you have to re-visit one, you are not a failure, you are just continuing your journey. Start, re-start or re-calibrate your relationship with food, one baby step at a time.

We thank you for allowing us to share our journeys and we wish you the best.

The Sis Sisters
Lisa (Bigg Sis) and Julia (Little Sis)

Recipes follow and of course there are countless terrific healthy cookbooks and blogs including ours – babystepstobetterhealth.com - out there waiting for you.

Baby Steps to Better Health / Recipes

Recipes!

The recipe section contains the following abbreviations to help you find recipes that meet you and your family's needs

(V) Vegan – no animal products whatsoever; if it is marked vegan, you can assume it is dairy free so you will not see DF on that recipe; for items like chocolate chips that come in both vegan and dairy versions, we assume you'll get vegan chips if that's what you're after

(DF) – Dairy free: no milk, cheese, butter, yogurt, etc. There may be eggs in a DF recipe but there will not be eggs in a (V) recipe. There may be other animal products, and there may be honey.

(GF) – Gluten free; if you are preparing meals for someone who is very sensitive to gluten, please be certain that you choose carefully when purchasing items such as oats, which are sold both gluten free and potentially not gluten free.

(DF, GF, or V Option) – This indicates that the recipe as we've written it is not dairy free or vegan, but we've included choices in parentheses that will allow you to very easily convert the recipe to meet your preferences.

While you will notice a preponderance of (V) dishes, we encourage you to adapt any of these recipes to suit your needs. We regularly explore recipes that have foods in them that we don't eat and simply change them around in our kitchens. This is how we cook – staying open to different kinds of recipes allows us to explore flavors and combinations we might not have otherwise considered. Take a look around; you just might surprise yourself.

Appetizers & Dips
ARTICHOKE DIP (VERY EASY & EASY) (GF/V)

VERY EASY:

1 jar (or can) of marinated artichoke hearts (after checking the label for unsavory ingredients);

Dump into good blender (or food processor);
Run until creamy;
Scrape into a pretty bowl and provided scooping devices.

Should you not have marinated artichoke hearts......

EASY:

3 cups of drained artichoke hearts
1 Tbsp. olive oil
1/2 tsp each of oregano & thyme (your option to include or sub basil or rosemary)
1 Tbsp. lemon juice (optional)
¼ – ½ tsp salt

Process until creamy.

Scrape into a pretty bowl and provide scooping devices.

BAJA HUMMUS (GF/V)
Inspired by Dreena Burton's Black Bean & Orange Hummus in *Eat, Drink, and Be Vegan*

2.5 c cooked black beans
1/4 c orange juice
3 Tbsp tahini (or nut butter of whatever kind you have)
1 large clove garlic
1 Tbsp olive oil
3 Tbsp red wine vinegar
3/4 tsp salt
1 tsp cumin
1/4 tsp chili powder (whatever kind you like)
1/3 c fresh parsley
1 tsp orange zest (zest before squeezing juice, trust me)

Throw all of your ingredients into a food processor and go to town. Stop a couple of times to scrape down bowl with spatula. Process until you get the consistency you like.

We love this slathered onto a whole wheat tortilla and covered with a whole mess of spinach and a few slices of avocado.

CHOCOLATE ALMOND BUTTER (GF/V)

3 cups roasted almonds
½ tsp salt
2 Tbsp. cocoa
1 Tbsp. maple syrup
A little time and patience... maybe another task in the kitchen to complete while doing this :-)

IF you are weaning a child from a very sugar-y breakfast or snack, then you may have to put a bit more sweetener in. My son loves this, but he is somewhat trained and does not often get sweets at the commercial level of sweet-ness, so he thought it was very yummy indeed. Taste as you go.

Roast almonds at 375 for about 10 minutes or until fragrant. It is quicker if you roast them on something that allows them to be spread out. If they are bunched up, shake them up every couple of minutes.
Place the almonds in the food processor with the S blade (the small metal guy that goes in the bottom).
Process until walls of almond crumbs are climbing up the side of your processor. Scrape it down and turn it back on. This is the patience piece. It takes about 12 minutes of processing to turn almonds into almond butter.
Once the almond butter is getting a bit MORE liquid than you want, add the cocoa and sweetener and process just to mix in.

If you want plain almond butter, just stop when the roasted almonds and salt reach the desired consistency. That's it!

DILLY SUNFLOWER CHEESE SPREAD (GF/V)
- adapted from Janet L. Doone's sprouted sunflower cheese[56]

1 c soaked sunflower seeds (soak them in water for at least an hour and rinse well)
1/4 c water
1 TBSP apple cider vinegar
juice from 1/2 to 1 lemon
1 small clove garlic
3/4 tsp salt
1 Tbsp chopped fresh dill (or herb of your choice or omit altogether)

The original recipe suggests rubbing the hulls off of the soaked sunflower seeds to ensure that the spread is more white than grey colored. I tried this for about a minute and found it tedious in the extreme. I decided instead to place the rinsed seeds on a paper towel and then place a second towel on top, rubbed a bit and then picked off the hulls that were identifiable. Not as thorough, but apparently it was enough. If you're okay with grey, I'd suggest skipping the hull concern altogether. Place all ingredients but water and dill in food processor. Add one half of the water and process. Add more water (by a few drops or a glug at a time) as needed to achieve good blending and a smooth texture. This can take some time – just let the thing grind away. The longer you let it go, the smoother your spread will be. When you've achieved the texture you like, scrape into bowl and mix in your dill. Serve on bread or crackers or on your sandwich, or in your pasta, or on your finger. Please don't eat your finger.

GARBANZORANGE HUMMUS (GF/V)

2.5 c cooked garbanzo beans
1/3 c orange juice
3 Tbsp tahini
1 small garlic clove
1 Tbsp olive oil
2 Tbsp red wine vinegar
3/4 tsp salt
1/2 tsp cumin
1/4 c parsley
1 tsp orange zest

Place all in food processor bowl. Go to it. Scrape down sides a couple of times. Run it until it's the consistency you like. Suggest to your little ones that maybe they'd like some chickpea (okay, so I called them tushies, cause you know the chickpea has a little bum on it and it cracks my kids up) hummus. Totally different reception. Still didn't win over my picky one, but she at least took a bite.

LEMONY ROASTED GARLIC HUMMUS (GF/V)

3 cups cooked and rinsed chickpeas (save the cooking water or canned water to use below)
6 cloves roasted garlic
1 tsp lemon zest
juice from 1 ½ lemons
4 Tbsp tahini
6 Tbsp water
1 tsp ground cumin
1 tsp salt (or to taste)
1 Tbsp olive oil (or your favorite)

Place all in food processor and beat the heck out of it. Mix a little before adding the water as it makes for less sloppage up the sides of the processor bowl, but of course you can always scrape down the sloppage. Depending on the softness of your chickpeas and your tahini, you may need to add a little extra water or oil. Get the hummus to a consistency that you like.Serve with crackers, pita bread, fresh veggies, salad – or turn some into an easy sauce Lemony Hummus Sauce.

NAVY BEAN HERB HUMMUS (GF/V)
– adapted from Dreena Burton's White Bean Hummus in *Eat, Drink and Be Vegan*

2 c cooked navy beans (cook until decidedly VERY soft, unless you like chunky hummus)
Juice of 1 small lemon
2 Tbsp tahini (or other unsweetened nut butter)
1 large clove garlic
2 Tbsp olive oil
2 Tbsp red wine vinegar
½ tsp mild (such as Dijon) mustard
½ tsp sea salt
black pepper to taste
water as needed
2 Tbsp chopped fresh thyme
¼ c chopped fresh basil
2 Tbsp chopped fresh parsley

Throw all ingredients except water and herbs in food processor. Go to it until desired consistency, adding tablespoons of water as required to achieve your hummusy heart's content. Pause periodically to scrape the bowl so all of the beans get through the blades. Add herbs at end and pulse a few times to blend without mutilating. (Wow. I may need to go get some right now. Just talking about this one makes me hungry.) Serve with whole wheat pitas, crackers, or a fresh baguette.

NUTTY GREENS DIP (GF/V)

Mix in the Vita Mix blender (or other powerful blender)

2 cups de-stemmed mustard leaves
4Tbsp. olive oil
1 &1/2 cup cooked white beans – rinsed and drained (1 can)
1/2 cup walnuts
1/2 cup raw cashews
1/2 tsp salt

Blend into smoothness, spreadable, dippable-ness.

Baby Steps to Better Health / Recipes: Appetizers & Dips

With the bite of mustard, this one is really good on a sandwich.

Admittedly, you may not have mustard greens around – however, the basic idea gives you the basis to veggify and/or herbify some bean mash into something healthy and delicious. Take the beans, nuts and oil in the above recipe, add some other veggies and spices, adjust for consistency and you will have expanded the repertoire for healthy lunch and snacks.

NUTTY LUNCH DIP (GF/V Option)

4 Tbsp peanut butter
4 Tbsp plain yogurt (I used almond yogurt)
1/2 tsp maple syrup
generous shake cinnamon

Ready for another miraculous cooking procedure? Put all those bits in a bowl and stir them thoroughly to make smooth yum. Adjust ingredients to taste. If it seems like a little more sweet would be good, try a little more cinnamon first; you may be surprised. When you've got it tasting the way you want, dip a few things in it. Let your inner five your old take control of the lunch plate. Pretend you don't already know what tastes good together; you just might find something new hiding in the guise of an old trusted and predictable vegetable. Nutty small bites for all!

ROASTED CHILI LIME NUTS (GF/V)
adapted from Shannon at A Cozy Place Called Home[57]

4 c nuts (Any kind is fine. I used almonds, salted peanuts, pecans, and walnuts.)
3 Tbsp coconut oil (melted) – original recipe is butter so that would work
3 Tbsp lime juice
1 ½ Tbsp chili powder
3 cloves garlic (pressed)
Salt: If you use salted nuts, don't add salt. I added 1/2 tsp because only the peanuts were salty.

Preheat oven to 350. Combine all ingredients but nuts in a small bowl and mix. Add nuts and stir
Pour out onto cookie sheet with edges. Make sure to scrape the extra off the bowl with a spatula
Bake approximately 15 – 20 minutes or until nuts are golden brown. Stir a couple of times in there for even coating and browning. Allow nuts to cool.

SMOKY BABA GHANOUSH (GF/ V)
- method and starting point borrowed from The Joy of Cooking

1 eggplant (mine was about 2 lbs, big and VERY purple, just beautiful)
1 Tbsp tahini
2 large cloves of garlic
½ lemon juiced
1 tsp salt
1/8 t chipotle pepper powder (you could also use an actual pepper, but be VERY sparing, you're going for the smokiness, not the heat, you could also use Liquid Smoke I imagine)

Preheat the oven to 400. Poke holes all over the eggplant with a fork. Roast the eggplant (and garlic cloves (skins on) in a roasting dish or on a baking sheet. Take the garlic out after about 15 minutes. Leave the eggplant in for about another 45. You're looking for very dark skin and more importantly, soft flesh. Allow eggplant to cool to handle it. Scoop the flesh of the eggplant away from the skin of the eggplant and place in a colander. When all the eggplant is in the colander, press down with a spoon or other flat utensil to squeeze the extra water out of the eggplant. The hard part is now over. Throw all of this with the other ingredients into the food processor. Blitz. Place in lovely bowl and garnish with olives. Serve to your generous mother who has been playing with your children for several hours… or to whomever you like.

SWEET ORANGE SUNFLOWER DIP (GF/ V)

1 c raw sunflower seeds soaked for at least 6 hours in 2 cups of water
zest from ½ – 1 orange. Zest is a little tart, so if you are wary, start with 1/2 and add more if you want
juice from 1 orange (was a bit less than 1/4 cup if you have juice in the fridge)
1 Tbsp maple syrup
1 tsp vanilla

Place all ingredients in food processor and run it for a few minutes until well combined. Scrape down the sides a few times to catch the errant seeds. Serve with fruit.

Bread Recipes
BLENDER BANANA BREAD (GF/V)

1 flax egg (1 Tbsp flax meal and 3 Tbsp water – mix and let sit for 5 – 10 minutes)
¼ c coconut oil
1/3 c milk of choice – I used homemade almond milk
2 ripe bananas
1 tsp vanilla extract
zest of 1 lemon (or sub ½ tsp lemon extract)
1 cup GF baking flour (I used Bob's Red Mill)
1/3 cup brown rice flour
1/3 cup buckwheat flour (you could probably sub other GF flours for these 2)
2 tsp baking powder
½ c sugar
¾ c chopped walnuts

Mix your flax egg if using (1 Tbsp freshly ground flax meal to 3 Tbsp cold water, stir and let sit)

While egg is setting…Pre-heat oven to 350. Lightly grease a loaf pan (I used coconut oil). Mix the last 6 ingredients in a bowl. Put the first 6 ingredients in the blender. Blend the wet ingredients on low until chunks are gone. Pour the wet into the dry ingredients and mix until incorporated. Pour into loaf pan. Bake at 350 for 45 – 55 minutes, or until toothpick comes out clean. Let cool for a bit before slicing or it will crumble and smush.

MIXED GRAIN BREAD (V)
– adapted from Anna Thomas' in *The Vegetarian Epicure*, p. 39.

2 c boiling water
1 Tbsp salt
3-4 Tbsp olive oil, divided
1 Tbsp molasses
1 c yellow corn meal
1 c rolled (old fashioned) oats
½ c lukewarm water
2 packages yeast (or 4 ½ tsp if you're not using packages)
3 c whole wheat flour
1 ½ c white whole wheat flour

Stir boiling water, salt, 2 T olive oil and molasses in large mixing bowl (or in bowl of stand mixer). Stir in corn meal and oats and let this mixture sit for AT LEAST 10 minutes. You're going for lukewarm – too warm and you'll kill the yeast later – but no pressure, and remember dense bread is still yummy. ;-) While the grains are cooling, dissolve the yeast into the warm water. Let sit while grains are cooling and then add yeasty water to grains. Stir in the whole wheat flour. Add the white whole wheat by 1/4 c measures until the dough becomes stiff and cohesive (tacky but not sticky or gooey).

If using a stand mixer, use the dough hook to knead the dough for at least 5 minutes. If kneading by hand, turn dough out onto lightly floured surface and knead for at least 5 minutes. If the dough becomes too sticky, add more flour. After at least five minutes of kneading, dough should be smooth and stretchy to the touch. Form a ball and place it in a large, oiled bowl. Turn the dough over so that it is oiled on all sides. Cover the bowl with a towel and leave it in a warm place to rise until doubled (around 1 ½ hours).

When the dough has doubled, punch it down and form it into two loaves. Place loaves on a baking sheet that has been oiled or lined with parchment paper. Preheat oven to 375 degrees. Let the loaves rise for about another ½ hour (until they've almost doubled). Just before putting bread in oven, slice down the middle with a sharp knife – just breaking the skin of the dough, not cutting the loaf into pieces. Bake in hot oven on middle rack for about 45 minutes. About half way through, brush the loaves with the reserved olive oil to encourage browning and olive oil goodness. You needn't use all the olive oil if it doesn't make sense – my measurement on this part was not measuring spoon aided.

Remove from oven when the crust feels firm and is slightly browned. Allow to cool on a wire rack for at least 15 minutes prior to slicing and devouring.

MULTIGRAIN BREAD WITH SUNFLOWER SEEDS (V)
- adapted from Deborah Madison[58]

The Sponge:

1 cup uncooked multigrain cereal (I used Bob's Red mill hot cereal, I've no idea if this is what she meant, but it worked)
1 ½ c hot water
1 c almond milk
2 ¼ tsp active dry yeast
1 c whole wheat flour

The Bread:

2 ½ tsp salt
2 Tbsp safflower oil (or as you like) plus extra for glazing
¾ c sunflower seeds
4 c whole wheat flour (I used 2 whole wheat and 2 white whole wheat as this was what I had)

Mix ingredients for the sponge in a bowl (If you have a stand mixer, use the bowl for it). Cover it (I used a clean dishtowel) and let sit for an hour. Your sponge should become bubbly and should smell, well, yeasty. Stir the sponge to release the air and add the salt, oil, and sunflower seeds. Begin stirring in the flour (move to stand mixer for this if you have one, if not no worries, totally doable by hand).

If using a mixer, switch to dough hook if you have one as you get down toward the end of the flour to add. When all flour is in, allow mixer to knead for a couple of minutes. If mixing by hand, stir flour in until it is too heavy to manage, then put the bread onto a lightly floured cutting board or counter and knead in the remaining flour by adding a little at a time and folding the bread dough over on itself until the dough is tacky but not wet or overly sticky.

Put dough in oiled bowl and allow to rise to double size, about an hour and a half (a warm but not HOT location will help this process). Push down the dough, divide into two and shape into loaves (I'm sure there are right ways to do this, I just fiddle with it until it looks loaf-ish. Place in oiled and floured 4 1/2 x 8 1/2 inch loaf pans and let rise again for about 45 minutes. About 25 minutes into this rise time, preheat your oven to 375.

Cut the top of the bread and brush the top with oil to glaze. Bake in the middle of the oven for about 45 minutes or until brown and awesome. Allow to cool for at least 15 minutes before serving to preserve the texture.

NO-FEAR WHOLE WHEAT BREAD (V)

2 cups coconut milk (or whatever you like)
3 Tbsp olive oil
1 Tbsp salt
3 Tbsp honey
2 Tbsp yeast
1/3 c warm (not hot) water
½ c oat bran (or wheat germ)
5 ½ to 6 c whole wheat flour

Heat milk to scalding. While heating, combine olive oil, salt, and honey in mixer bowl (if using a stand mixer) or large bowl if working by hand. Allow ingredients to sit for at least 10 minutes to cool to lukewarm. While cooling, add yeast to warm water and allow to dissolve and become frothy. Add to lukewarm mixture in bowl. Add bran and 3 c flour. Stir with wooden spoon or stand mixer until batter is incorporated. Add more flour by half cups until dough is too stiff to stir properly. Proceed according to your method below.

Stand Mixer: Change to dough hook. Add additional flour if necessary to bring dough to point of being only slightly sticky and forming a ball on the hook. Continue to knead with dough hook for 5-10 minutes, until dough becomes smooth and elastic.

Manual Prep: Turn dough onto floured board or countertop, adding more flour as necessary to achieve dough that is slightly sticky but not wet. Knead for at least five minutes by pushing dough to flatten and folding it back in on itself. Knead until dough is smooth and elastic.

ALL TOGETHER NOW:
Place dough into large oiled bowl. Turn dough over once so that the whole dough ball is lightly coated with oil. Place in warm spot with clean cloth over the bowl and allow to rise for an hour. Punch the dough down and allow to rise for another hour Knead a few times and shape the dough into 2 loaves.

Place in oiled loaf pans, cover and allow to rise for 45 minutes or until dough is nearly doubled. If you are allowing to rise in the oven, remove after half an hour to preheat oven. Bake for 45 minutes at 375. Loaves should brown a bit and feel like great bread (you'll know). Your house will smell FANTASTIC for most of this process. Who needs air freshener? Just bake some bread. Remove from oven and allow to cool in pan for a couple of minutes. Then remove to wire rack.

Despite the overwhelming temptation, please don't cut into your bread for at least 15 minutes or you will squish up the insides and make them less tasty. Notice I only say less, and less tasty than awesome is still pretty darned good.

PEPPERY CHEEZE BREAD (V)
- inspired by Peppered Cheese Bread in Deborah Madison's *Vegetarian Cooking for Everyone* (yes, you should get it)

1 1/3 c warm water
2 ¼ tsp active dry yeast
1 ½ tsp salt
1 tsp fine ground pepper (I used white pepper in a foolish attempt to hide it)
1 tsp red pepper flakes
1 beaten egg (I used flax)
4 c white whole wheat flour
1/2 c sunflower cheese (see recipe in sides section)

Pour warm water into large bowl (or the bowl of a stand mixer) and stir in the yeast. Allow to sit about 10 minutes or until slightly foamy. Add salt, pepper, pepper flakes, all but 1 Tbsp of the egg and all but one cup of the flour. Mix or stir until smooth. Add sunflower cheese. Mix or stir to incorporate. For stand mixer, change over to dough hook and knead for about 5 minutes. If mixing by hand, add the rest of the flour and knead by hand to incorporate. Continue to knead by hand (folding the dough in on itself repeatedly and pushing it flat) for about 5 minutes. Put the dough in an oiled bowl, turn over once, cover and place in warm spot to rise for about an hour (until doubled).

Push the dough down, turn it out onto the counter or a floured surface. Shape into a ball. Cover until doubled, another 45 minutes to an hour. Preheat to 375 during the last 15 minutes of rising. Slash an X on the top, brush with olive oil. Bake on a preheated stone or pan for 45 minutes and cool on a rack. Allow to cool at least 10 minutes before you cut in and devour it.

VEGAN CREAM BISCUITS (V)
– adapted from happyherbivore.com[59]

2 c whole wheat pastry flour
5 tsp baking powder
¼ tsp salt
4 Tbsp Not So Sour Cream (in sauces section)
2 Tbsp olive oil
1 c non-dairy milk

Preheat oven to 400. Stir together dry ingredients. Put in food processor, add NSSC and olive oil. Pulse until the clumps of creaminess and fat are not clumping. Return to bowl and stir in non-milk. Drop in ¼ c blobs onto greased baking sheet (or use parchment). Bake in oven on low rack for 15 minutes. Remove from oven and slather with whatever floats your biscuit boat. We like ours with Date Cream (in breakfast section)

Breakfast Recipes

APPLE DRIZZLE (GF/V) (for pancakes / French toast / hot cereal)

Let's be honest, pancakes are yummy, but that's mostly because they are a vehicle for maple syrup or honey. Maple syrup and honey are both natural, right? That's good, right?

Well….I wish they were not still sugar, but chemistry tells us that they are both still sugar with the negative physiological impact (albeit minus some leftover chemicals from processing and nasty effects on the planet).

So here, and under Date Cream are other options for sweetening breakfast a little more gently…

Apples (I used 1 large and 1 small).
1 – 5 Tbsp water
1 tsp maple syrup
pinch of salt

Core and chop apples in sizes appropriate to the estrogen level of your blender. (My blender is a Vita Mix…. very high estrogen level! I leave skins on – more nutrition and a speck of color ☺. Add about a Tablespoon of water and start the blender on low. Add water as needed to get the stuff spinning and pourable. To the pourable apple mixture I added 1 teaspoon of maple syrup and a pinch of salt.

Pour on many things.

BEAR-Y GOOD OATS (GF if using GF oats/V)
- inspired by the bear who came to eat sunflower seeds from the birdfeeder in Little Sis' backyard.

2 c rolled oats
2 c almond milk (or whatever kind you like)
zest of one lemon
raw sunflower seeds
berries

Place oats, milk, and zest in bowl or jar overnight to soak (the lemon zest was Big Sis' idea). In the morning, spoon out some of that deliciousness in a bowl and top with sunflower seeds and berries of your choosing. Bear-y Good!

Baby Steps to Better Health / Recipes: Breakfast

BREAKFAST ICE CREAM (GF/V)

3-4 frozen bananas
1/2 ripe avocado
3 cups deep greens (or more if you can get away with it)
frozen berries to top of blender container
1 soup spoon honey (opt – we use if the berries are tart, i.e. raspberries)
non-dairy milk (we used coconut) until blend ability (usually 1.5 cups for us) or some other liquid of your choosing

If you a power blender, this is very easy. Mix and go! If you have a standard blender or an aging power blender you don't wish to replace, start with the liquid and the non-frozen ingredients, and then add the frozen ingredients slowly. This makes a lot of breakfast ice cream, which is awesome, because if you have leftovers you can freeze and pack in a lunch. Breakfast ice cream. THAT's living.

BUCKWHEAT BREAKFAST BOWL (GF/V)

Buckwheat is not actually wheat – it is a seed from a non-wheat plant that is somewhat pyramidal in shape. For this recipe you want the actual seeds, not flour.

1 handful of buckwheat groats per person
1 handful raw sunflower seeds per person

Place in a bowl and cover with about 2" of water. Cover the bowl and let it sit overnight.
Rinse until the water runs clear the next morning – it will look a little cloudy and slimy. Serve as is or add a little almond, soy or cow's milk along with some raisins or chopped dates, nuts, or other fruit, a little cinnamon adds some sweetness as well.

BUTTERMILK WHOLE WHEAT PANCAKES

If you use a cast iron pan for pancakes, place it in the oven at 350 to warm. Place on the stove over medium low heat when ready to use.

1 cup whole wheat or white whole wheat flour
1 cup oats
1 tsp. salt
1 Tbsp. baking powder
1 & 3/4 cups buttermilk
2 eggs
2 Tbsp. oil
1 tsp vanilla (optional)
handful raw cashews (optional but very tasty!)

Baby Steps to Better Health / Recipes: Breakfast 134.

I usually make 1 & 1/2 or 2 times this recipe so there will be leftovers to freeze. Mix dry. Mix wet. Mix the 2. Pour small amounts into heated pan, flip when bubbles are present and edges look dry, eat.

CHOCOLATE ALMOND BUTTER (GF/V) or 'Buttella – a hybrid of Butter & Nutella'

2 ½ - 3 c roasted almonds (roast your own for 10 minutes at 375)
½ tsp salt
2 Tbsp cocoa
1 Tbsp maple syrup (can sub agave if you like)
A little time and patience... maybe another task in the kitchen to complete while doing this :-)

Put the roasted almonds and salt in the food processor, let it run until you have almond butter which is a bit too wet to put on toast or bread. This will take a long time and will require some scraping down occasionally to keep things spinning. It can take 10 - 15 minutes to reach smooth stage. Add the cocoa and sweetener and spin a bit more.

CHOCO-NANA PANCAKES (DF option/V option)

2 c whole wheat flour
½ c wheat germ
½ c white whole wheat flour
4-5 Tbsp cocoa powder (we used five and it was a deep dark choco flavor)
4 tsp baking powder
1 ½ tsp baking soda
1 ½ tsp salt
3 eggs (I used flax)
3 Tbsp oil (I used safflower)
2 extremely ripe bananas
2 ½ c milk (I used almond milk)

If you can heat your pans ahead of time (with an oven timer), do that as it makes for less sticking and more even cooking. If not, put them in the oven before you do anything and set the heat to 325 or so. If you're mixing flax eggs and didn't do it the night before, do it now before you do everything else. Mix dry ingredients in a large bowl. Mash bananas in a smaller bowl. Mix oil into the bananas or one of the other wet ingredients. Add wet ingredients to dry ingredients and stir until you don't see any more dry flour or flour clumps. Let the batter rest for at least 10 minutes. Pour batter into pans using a ¼ c measure.

If you're really feeling decadent, add a few chocolate chips to them while they cook (my kids like to SEE what's in them, so I don't mix into the batter), and if you're like me and you desire a little texture in your life, throw some nuts in too (I used pecans). Wait for bubbles and relatively dry edges, then flip. Cook a minute or two longer and serve piping hot. The kids had their first with syrup and then switched to strawberry jam (which is great with chocolate, by the way). I enjoyed mine with a little bit of coconut butter and a splash of syrup.

DARK CHOCOLATE STEEL CUT OATS (GF/V)

adapted from Kathy Hester's *The Vegan Slow Cooker*[60]

2 c steel cut oats
8 c water (or nut milk, or cow's milk)
6 Tbsp cocoa powder (you can adjust to your own preference)
3 tsp vanilla
4 Tbsp maple syrup

Oil the crock of your slow cooker (I used coconut oil and wow is that always good with chocolate). Add all the ingredients. Give a little stir. Cook on low for 6-8 hours. Stir before you try to tempt anyone with it – it doesn't look particularly appealing at first sight. A good stir will make it look like, well, dark chocolate steel cut oats.

DATE CREAM (DF/V Option) - (for pancakes or French toast, or a sweetener for hot cereal, or to sweeten up whoever might be grumpy in the morning)

Place whole pitted dates in your blender (I used a Vita Mix, you may need a powerful blender for this) up to about the 1 cup line.

Pour almond, soy or cow (I used unsweetened almond) milk to cover

Whip it good. (Any DEVO fans out there?)

Seek the creaminess level that your heart tells you is right Grasshopper…
i.e. add a little more milk of your choice until you get a consistency that you think will be moist enough for whatever you are putting it on.

I was originally planning to add just a little maple syrup or honey to this mix, but then I tasted it. WOW! I will have to be careful not to just make this and eat 3 pounds of it, because dates are not cheap and 3 pounds of anything will show up on me somewhere… and usually NOT where I would have directed the placement of extra flesh.

FABU VEGAN PANCAKES (V with non V options)

1.5c whole wheat flour
.5c rolled oats
2tsp baking powder

1tsp baking soda
1tsp salt
nutmeg to taste
4Tbsp oil
1Tbsp maple syrup
2 flax eggs (or 2 chicken eggs)
2 c non-dairy milk (2c buttermilk)

Place cast iron skillet in oven at 325 and warm. In large bowl, combine and stir dry ingredients. In small bowl, combine eggs and oil. Pour egg/oil into dry ingredients. Add milk one cup at a time, stirring gently and watching the batter for consistency. If you like thicker pancakes, you may want to use a little less milk. Stir gently to mix dry with wet. Let rest for at least 10 minutes. Drop batter into pre-warmed skillet by 1/4c measure. If you're feeling extra decadent drop a few chocolate chips onto the cooking pancake. It only take a few to make a five year old think something REALLY special is happening. Watch the edges for firming. Watch for bubbles. Flip and cook until just barely cooked through.

GRANOLA (GF if using GF oats / V option)
Recipe adapted from Ruth Yaron's *Super Baby Food*

Pre-heat oven to 350

Spread 5 cups oats in a 9×13 dish (I usually do 2 dishes at the same time)

Heat the oats for 10 minutes

While the oats are heating, mix:

1/2 cup oil
1/3 cup honey, maple syrup or a combo
1 teaspoon vanilla
(for each batch: if making 2 batches at once I mix this in 2 separate measuring cups so I can add one to each dish of 5 cups oats)

Chop or break one cup of nuts for each batch

When oats are warm add the nuts plus:

1 cup unsweetened coconut (available at some groceries in bulk or at a health food store)
1 tsp cinnamon
plus one oil/sweetener mixture to each pan

Stir. Bake, mixing granola after 10 minutes and then after every 5 minutes for a total of 25 – 30 minutes, or until brown. Let cool. Keep in airtight container

HEARTY, HEALTHY HOT CEREAL AKA **Warm Bowl of Yum (GF/V)**

5 cups liquid: I use 2 ½ water and 2 ½ almond milk
1 c oats
1 c quinoa
1 c ground walnuts (you can certainly try other nuts, but walnuts really seem to thicken this and they are not very noticeable either ;-)
1 tsp salt (optional)
1-2 tsp allspice / or 1 Tbsp cinnamon (optional)
toppings like raisins, honey, more nuts, maple syrup, etc.

Bring your liquid and salt, if using, to a boil. Be careful! Almond milk is the wallflower of boilers. It waits and waits and then suddenly gets inspired, leaps into the fray, jumps out of the pan and into the saucer under your burner there to create a rather ghastly smell and even ghastlier mess. Do not step away from the stove until you're at a safe simmer!

Once it boils, toss in your quinoa, turn down to a simmer and cover. Let simmer about 10
minutes and then boil again Baby! Toss in the oatmeal, turn down to low and cover. Let simmer about 5 minutes. While it is simmering, grind your walnuts. I am blessed with a Vita-Mix which is a noisy but effective way to grind nuts. Stir in the ground nuts and cook covered for a few minutes or until the oats are tender and the quinoa is tender. Schplop into bowls with your favorite schplopper, top with your favorite toppers and enjoy!

MAPLE CASHEW BUTTER (GF/V)

1 ½ c raw cashews
¼ c maple syrup
1 tsp vanilla
4 Tbsp water

Place all in food processor and turn on. Check back periodically and scrape down the sides until well incorporated and creamy. Serve over your favorite pancakes, French toast, nut butter sandwiches or carrots / apples, etc.

MOMMA'S MULTIGRAIN THANKSGIVING PANCAKES (DF & V Options)

1½ c whole wheat flour
½ c all purpose flour
½ c corn meal
½ c spelt or buckwheat flour
3 tsp baking powder
1 ½ tsp baking soda
1 ½ tsp salt
nutmeg to taste
3 eggs (I used flax eggs)
3 c butter milk or soured milk (I used soured almond milk)
6 T oil (I used canola)
cooked sweet potato cut into small bites
handful of dried fruit
handful of pecans (toasted if you're really going for it)

When I make pancakes, I mix the dry ingredients and prepare the flax eggs (1T flax meal to 3T water for one egg, in bowl, in fridge) the night before. I can't speak for everyone, but I am hungry when I wake up and I don't like waiting TOO long for breakfast. I also put my pans in the oven and set it pre-heat them before we get up because I'm fussy like that.Upon rising, I task whichever munchkin is up with mixing the dry ingredients while I whisk the oil and flax eggs together. Add wet ingredients to dry ingredients and stir until just combined. I then remind wakeful and hungry munchkins that we must let the batter rest. While resting, I gather my "flavors" (sweet potato pre-cooked and cut into small pieces, toasted pecans and dried fruit). Remove warmed pans from oven and turn on heat on stove to bring to temp. After at least 10 minutes of resting, pour batter using a 1/4c measure onto med warm pan. Add mix-ins (I find it takes surprisingly little, especially of things like craisins, to get the flavor without overwhelming). I realize many people mix in their flavors, but I prefer adding them to the pancakes once in the pan. This way the fruits get a little brown edge and you can SEE what you are eating, and you're more likely to get all the bits in one bite – yes, I am that particular. Flip when pancake edges are firm, and there are a few bubbles in the batter.

OPEN SUMMER SAMMIE BREKKIE (V)

whole grain bread (I used Ezekial)
ripe avocado
sliced tomato
chopped fresh basil
sprinkle salt & pepper

Toast bread if you prefer
Spread the avocado on the bread.
Place tomato slices on top of avocado.
Sprinkle with basil, salt, and pepper.

PECAN PANCAKES (DF/V option)

This is simply a riff on my usual pancake concoction. I've left out the buckwheat this time as the more adventurous of my two was expressing objections, thought I'd cut him a break.

2 c whole wheat flour
½ c all purpose flour
½ c corn meal
3 tsp baking powder
1 ½ tsp salt
1 ½ tsp baking soda
nutmeg to taste
3 eggs (I used flax)
6 Tbsp oil
3 c buttermilk or soured milk (I used almond)
a couple of handfuls of pecans, toasted if you've time and broken or cut into large chunks

Mix the dry. Mix the wet. Mix together. After all the mixing, just prepare pancakes as usual.

QUICK SWEET POTATO BREKKIE (GF/V)

leftover sweet potato (mine was baked and then broiled w/coconut oil and salt)
leftover quinoa
shredded unsweetened coconut
chopped pecans
drizzle maple syrup

Open the sweet potato and spoon some leftover quinoa over the potato halves. Warm briefly in the microwave and then top with the other ingredients.

SIMPLE OVERNIGHT STEEL CUT OATS (GF if using GF oats/ V option)

oil for pot
2 cups steel cut oats
8 cups liquid – I mixed mine half water, half almond milk
cinnamon or nutmeg to taste

VERY lightly oil the bowl of the Crock Pot. Add ingredients. Stir. Cook for 7-8 hours on low. When you open the lid, it may not look like yummy oatmeal, but this is a result of the long low cook. Give it a stir, and voila, there's your hot oatmeal, ready to go. Serve with preferred oatmeal toppings. Here's where you say: "THAT'S IT?!" And I say, "Yes, that's it." Many people like to cook apples, dried fruit, nuts, whatever, in with their oatmeal. We tend to like the texture that these items add when put in individual bowls in the morning. This also allows for more individual choice (pretty much a necessity with two five year olds). Delish.

A Note On Crock Pots: There are a variety of Crock Pots and slow cookers on the market and you can spend very little or a whole lot. There are also LOTS of people who have Crock Pots in the back of their cabinets that they don't use. Ask around; see what you can dig up. But wait, you say, the new ones have timer functions and all sorts of other cool features. To which I say, yes, they do and you will pay for it. Unless you're planning on doing a WHOLE lot of Crock Pot cooking (which I do), I'd like to suggest that you consider my ridiculously simple solution: the cheapest Crock Pot you can find with a four dollar wall timer. Worked like a charm. So if you have an old Crock Pot, your Aunt Martha has an old Crock Pot, or if you're lucky like me and attended a White Elephant holiday party with a bunch of younger folks who couldn't imagine the utility of a Crock Pot, slap that timer on there and you have breakfast in bed (because you could actually cook it in your room, you know) ready to go. Hot Diggity!

SWEET POTATO AND RICE BOWL (GF/V)

- per person recipe and of course the size of your people may necessitate portion changes!

1/2 – 1 cooked sweet potato (I always leave skin on)
1/2 – 1 cup cooked brown rice
1 tsp. ground cinnamon
1 - 2 Tbsp. raisins (optional but highly recommended)
1 - 2 Tbsp. pecans or walnuts (optional but highly recommended)
A splash of milk of whatever kind for those who like moist (optional)

Place together in a bowl. You can chop the sweet potato if you wish -- I just cut it as I ate and mixed in the other stuff.

Re-heat and eat. Very satisfying, healthy and delicious – and it's really already made if you cook the potatoes and rice the night before!

SWEET POTATO / APPLE / OAT NUCLEAR INCIDENT (GF/V Option)

1 – 2 sweet potatoes
1 - 2 apples
1 cup oats (I do not use quick oats – but they should be fine)

1 ¼ cups milk of your choice (I used unsweetened almond)
1 tsp vanilla
1 tsp – 1 Tbsp cinnamon (I use a lot because it lends sweetness without sugar and is so darn good!)
handful of chopped walnuts
optional: sweetener, raisins, other nuts, broccoli (just kidding)

Chop the sweet potatoes small. Place them in the microwave in a large bowl for a minute or two while chopping the apple. Add the apple to the bowl and nuke again for a minute. Add the oats, milk, vanilla, cinnamon, and walnuts and stir. Nuke for a minute and then stir again.

You can stop and eat this now if you like crunchier / more raw oats or you can nuke it again, but don't go more than a minute at a time – or even 45 seconds until you see how your microwave does so that it doesn't boil over the top. You can also add more milk or water if you want your oats softer.

Add any optional delights! Taste before sweetening as the cinnamon and apple might just do it for you!

VEGGIES 'N' OATS (GF/V)

bowl of oatmeal & leftover sweet potatoes (cooked to your preference; I like my oats decidedly underdone)
1 stalk celery, chopped and cooked with the oats
handful of fresh spinach or other mild green, chopped
palmful of raisins
sprinkle of grated coconut
handful of walnuts
splash of coconut milk (or your preference)

Prepare oatmeal with celery added.
Mix in everything else

WHOLE WHEAT BLUEBERRY PANCAKES (V)

3 c white whole wheat flour
1 c rolled oats
3 tsp baking powder
1 tsp baking soda
½ tsp salt
2 Tbsp coconut sugar (or whatever dry kind you use)
fresh ground nutmeg to taste
6 Tbsp coconut oil

½ c applesauce
1 banana, mashed
3 ½ c coconut milk (or whatever kind you like)
fresh blueberries as desired

Mix dry ingredients (through sugar). Add wet ingredients except for the milk, use a fork or a pastry cutter to blend in. Add milk and stir to combine. Let rest for 10 minutes. When your resting time (10 minutes) is up, pour batter into warm-hot pans. Add fresh blueberries by plopping them onto the pancakes in whatever ratio works for you. Wait for bubbles and flip.

We suggest serving with maple cashew butter (in this section).

Desserts & Sweets

Be forewarned that some of these recipes may not seem sweet to you. The level of sugar to which you are accustomed sort of dictates how sweet you expect dessert or a 'sweet' to be. As you work on lowering the amount of sugar and sweeteners you eat you will find deep satisfaction with less sugar than you are used to. ☺

ALMOND JOY BROWNIES (GF/V)
The Brownie – adapted from Sarah at Gazing In's Sweet Potato Fudgy Brownies[61]

¼ c coconut oil
2/3 c unsweetened cocoa powder or raw cacao if you're feeling spendy
1 c gluten free rolled oats blitzed in food processor until flour like
¼ tsp baking powder
¼ tsp salt
1 c coconut sugar
2/3 c sweet potato puree (baked sweet potato in food processor with enough water to create baby foodish consistency – add water SLOWLY so as not to overshoot)
1 Tbsp ground flax meal + 3 Tbsp water (AKA flax egg)
1 ½ tsp vanilla

Preheat Oven to 350. Melt coconut oil and add cocoa, stirring to create smooth, silky chocolate that you should not eat. Combine oat flour, baking powder and salt in small bowl. Combine coconut sugar, sweet potato puree, flax egg and vanilla in medium or larger bowl and whisk until smooth. Add chocolate. Stir to combine. Add dry ingredients (if you're still holding a whisk, now is the time to switch to a spoon, unless you're trying to create an "Oh no, I have so much brownie batter stuck in my whisk, however will I get it off…. slurp" kind of scenario. Not that I've ever done that.

Add a handful or so of your favorite chocolate chips. Scoop into oiled square baking dish. Bake for 35-40 minutes. Look for typical brownie crackling on top and a slightly firm feel in the middle of the pan (that second test is only for those of us in the asbestos fingers crowd). You can try the toothpick test, but these are fudgy, and will not likely come out totally clean. So just look for not wet, mostly clean. Remove and allow to cool in the pan.

The Topping

2 c shredded unsweetened coconut
16 whole raw almonds

Place coconut in food processor. Turn on and let it run, run, run. You're going to let it go so long that the coconut is going to turn into a liquid. Stop it occasionally and scrape the sides of the bowl so all of the coconut gets transformed into superific coconut butter. When the contents of the bowl are shiny, let it run a couple more minutes and then place in a container you can put a lid on so you can save the leftover and put it on your toast, in your oatmeal.... yes, the options are mind-boggling. When the brownies have cooled a little (you don't have to let them cool completely), spread the coconut butter on top in whatever amount makes sense to you.

I tried to show a little restraint because I wanted the chocolate flavor to prevail. If your coconut butter has hardened, gently warm it a little to soften. Place almonds on top – I did a one whole almond per brownie ratio, to get that crunch that I used to love in the Almond Joy, but I think chopped almonds would make for a nice effect as well.

ALMOND LEMON JOTS (GF/DF)
- adapted from Detoxinista's Frosted Almond Sugar Cookie recipe[62]

2 c almond flour
¼ cup coconut oil, softened
¼ cup honey
1 – 2 tsp. lemon zest (I say the more the better!)
½ teaspoon vanilla extract
¼ teaspoon salt

Frosting:

2 tablespoons coconut oil, softened
2 tablespoons raw honey
1 tsp lemon zest
pinch of salt

Preheat oven to 350F. In a medium bowl, mix together cookie ingredients. Drop by Tablespoon-ful onto a baking sheet, lined with a Silpat or parchment paper. Bake for about 8 minutes at 350F, or until the edges turn golden brown. Allow to cool on the pan for 10 minutes, then transfer to a wire rack to cool completely. For the frosting, cream together the coconut oil, honey, lemon zest and salt, until well combined. If the coconut oil starts to melt (it melts at temperatures above 76 degrees), briefly place the mixture in the fridge to help it set.

Frost the cooled cookies, and let them set in the fridge for a more solid-frosting.

APPLE OAT MUFFINS
Adapted from Average Betty's Oatmeal Apple Muffins[63]

1 cup oats
1 cup white whole wheat flour (that's what I used – haven't tried whole wheat)
1 tsp baking powder
1 tsp cinnamon
1/2 tsp baking soda

1/2 tsp salt
1/2 cup brown sugar
2/3 cup nuts
3/4 cup buttermilk
1/4 cup canola (or other oil you like)
1 large egg
1 tsp vanilla (I always go a little heavy on the vanilla)
1 large apple, chopped and seeded (I always leave the skin on)

Mix dry ingredients. Mix wet ingredients except apple. Mix dry and the wet and then fold in the apples! Pour into cupcake paper lined muffin pans and bake at 325 degrees for 20 minutes.

AWESOME OATIE BARS   (GF – if using GF oats/V)

1/2 c cashews
1/2 c almonds
1 c dried dates
1/3 c pumpkin seeds
juice of 1 lemon
1/4 c peanut butter (or other nut butter)
1 c raw oatmeal (approximately to taste)
2 Tbsp chocolate chips (just enough to make it a treat)

Put nuts in food processor and run until fine. Add pumpkin seeds, dates, lemon juice and peanut butter. Process until dough forms a large sticky ball (if ball isn't forming, add another splash of lemon or a tiny bit more nut butter).

Remove ball and place in large bowl. Add oats a little at a time (I did 1/3 c scoops) and mix into dough. I found bare hands to be the easiest (albeit messiest) way to do this. I used a cup of oats, but you may prefer a little more for less stickiness or less for more fruitiness. Mix in chocolate chips. Place plastic wrap in the bottom of a small baking dish (mine was square) and pat down until evenly distributed. Place in freezer for at least 1/2 hour. Cut into squares or bars depending on the size of snack you prefer to have available. We cut our square baking pan full into 16 pieces. Not too big for the kids, small enough to be negligible for the adults. The name of the dish comes from my son. "What do you think we should call them, buddy?" "Awesome Bars." I added the "oatie" to be marginally descriptive. Delish!

BALSAMIC STRAWBERRY PIE (GF/V Options)

1.5 pounds strawberries, hulled and sliced
1 Tbsp balsamic
1 Tbsp sugar

1 baked pie crust / tart crust / crust type thing of your preference/dietary needs
yogurt for drizzling (opt)

Mix strawberries, balsamic and sugar.
Let them sit for at least an hour
Spoon strawberries into cooled baked crust-type-thing-of-your-choice
Drizzle yogurt (sweetened or not) over the top very lightly

CHICKPEA CHOCOLATE CHIP BISCUITS (GF/V)
- makes 3 dozen biscuits

4 c gluten free oats, divided
1 ½ tsp baking soda
½ tsp salt
1 tsp cream of tartar (opt)
1 ripe banana
1 can (or 1 ½ c soaked) chickpeas (drained, rinsed)
½ c melted coconut oil
½ c maple syrup
1 tsp vanilla
¼ c coconut sugar (or other solid sugar)
½ c chopped toasted pecans
½ c semi-sweet or dark chocolate chips
¼ c unsweetened shredded coconut

Preheat oven to 350. Measure 2 c rolled oats into food processor and process until flour-like. Move to large bowl and add baking soda, salt, and cream of tartar. Place banana, chickpeas, coconut oil, maple syrup, vanilla, and sugar into food processor and process until chickpeas are completely ground and mixture is incorporated. It will be quite wet. Add wet to dry. Stir to combine. Add remaining 2 c rolled oats. Stir to mix. Add pecans, chips, and coconut. Stir to mix.
Scoop onto cookie sheet (greased or lined with parchment) using a cookie scoop if you've got one or two soup spoons if you don't. Flatten a bit with fingers or spoon and bake for 16-21 minutes. Look for some browning around the edges. Let cool on the tray for two minutes. Remove to wire racks to cool completely – and be sure to eat one warm.

BUCKWHEAT CHIPPERS (GF/V)
- inspired by Jordan's Buckwheat Chocolate Chip Cookies[64]

2 c buckwheat flour
1 ½ tsp baking soda
½ tsp salt
1/3 c canola oil (or whatever kind you like)

1/3 c applesauce
2/3 c maple syrup
1 tsp vanilla
heaping ½ c semi-sweet chocolate chips (I used minis to ensure choc in each bite and because, let's face it, they're cute)
½ c chopped pecans

Preheat oven to 350. Mix flour, baking soda and salt in large bowl. Mix wet ingredients in smaller bowl. Add wet to dry and stir. The dough will be wetter and easier to mix than traditional chocolate chip cookie dough. Don't be alarmed. The dough will also be considerably darker than you might expect. Again, it will all be okay.

Add chips and nuts (and whatever else your tribe prefers in such things) and stir gently to distribute. Plop onto parchment or greased baking sheets. I confess to using an official cookie dough scoop for such things (my Christmas baking requirements justified this little gem), but use whatever method you usually use with drop cookies. After filling the tray (I got 12-15 per tray), squash the tops a little as they will not spread the way higher fat cookies do. Bake for 6-9 minutes. Mine took 9, but my oven is wacky. Judge doneness by touching the cookie gently.
When it feels like a cookie and not a squishy ball, they're done. Allow to cool on the pan briefly for cleaner liftoff. Move to wire rack to continue cooling after you've eaten some while they're warm because you simply must eat some while they're warm.

CELEBRATION KRISPIES (GF/V)
- inspired by Dreena Burton's Nicer Krispie Squares in *Eat, Drink & Be Vegan* and Toffifay

½ c nut butter (I mixed almond and peanut as that's what I had)
½ c maple syrup
¼ tsp salt
1 ½ tsp vanilla extract
4 cups rice crisp cereal (I used Barbara's Bakery Brown Rice Crisps Cereal, but you could ABSOLUTELY use other cereals. I've used many different kinds of cereal in these kinds of bars and they all work – just go with what works for you)
1/3 – ½ c hazlenuts, rough chopped (this is part of the Toffifay magic)
¼ – 1/3 c dark chocolate chips (vegan if you want vegan!)
2 Tbsp chia seeds (totally optional, just threw them in for a little nutrition boost)

Line an 8 x 8 or a 9 x 11 with parchment paper – or lightly oil. Choose the size of the pan based on your preference. The square pan will give you thicker Krispie bars. Combine the nut butter, maple syrup, salt and vanilla in a saucepan on low-medium heat. Stir occasionally as ingredients melt and combine. A little bubbling is okay, but nothing crazy. Turn down if need be.

While the mixture is heating, put cereal, nuts, chocolate chips and chia seeds in a large bowl. When mixture is melted and combined, pour it over dry ingredients. Stir gently but with some haste as it will get harder to get everything to combine as the wet ingredients cool off. Stir until combined. Spoon into pan and gently press down. Stick in fridge to cool completely before cutting.

COCOANUTTY GOOD BARS (GF/V)
- adapted from Leslie's Bad But Good Bars in Dreena Burton's *Eat, Drink & Be Vegan*[65]

1 c nuts (I used salted cashews and sunflower seeds)
1 generous c oats, chopped slightly in food processor or with a knife
1/2 c unsweetened shredded coconut
2 T cocoa powder
1/3 c maple syrup
3 T coconut oil (melted)
1 c non-dairy chocolate chips (or regular if you don't care about that)
2/3 c extra firm tofu
1 t vanilla extract
2 T peanut butter (or whatever nut butter you prefer)

Combine first 6 ingredients (through coconut oil) in large bowl and mix until combined. The mixture will be crumbly, but should hold together when pressed. Scrape mixture into pan (I used a nonstick springform pan as that's what was in the beach house, and I was going for a birthday cake look. The original recipe suggests an 8 inch square lined with parchment. Press mixture down evenly.

Melt chocolate chips however you like (double boiler, bowl over pot, or microwave). Combine chips and remaining ingredients in food processor and process until smooth. Scrape out onto base layer and spread evenly. Place in fridge for at least two hours to allow chocolate to set.

Cut as you like (squares if you're reasonable, slices if it's a party) and serve. We had ours with a variety of ice creams (dairy and non-dairy).

CRANBERRY APPLE PECAN CRUNCH (GF/V)
– significantly adapted from Cherry Apple Pecan Crisp in *Hay Day Country Market Cookbook*

Fruit

8 cups thinly sliced tart apples (no I don't peel and I used Pink Lady)
¾ c dried cranberries
1/3 c fresh squeezed orange juice
¼ c coconut sugar (or your preferred sweetener)

Crunch

1 c rolled oats
¼ c chickpea flour (you can use whatever flour you prefer OR use more oats)
½ c coconut sugar (or your favorite solid sweet)
1 ½ tsp cinnamon
¼ tsp fresh ground nutmeg
8 Tbsp coconut oil (cold is ideal)
1 ½ c pecans (we toasted ours – WOW), chopped coarsely

Preheat oven to 350. Lay apples in rectangular baking dish (mine was the classic large glass variety). Sprinkle cranberries on, trying to distribute somewhat evenly. Add sugar to OJ and stir.
Drizzle over fruit, attempting vaguely even distribution. If you prefer, you can mix all of these together in a bowl and then put in pan, but I had little hands that needed occupying and she really enjoyed adding it to the pan in stages. Set the fruit aside.

Place dry ingredients through the nutmeg in a food processor and pulse a couple of times to mix. Add the coconut oil and process until incorporated and crumbly. Stir in pecans and pour the mixture over the waiting fruit. You can add a few raw oats to the top for texture. Bake until lightly browned and fruit juices bubble up around the edges 40-45 minutes. Cool for at least 10 minutes before serving.

CRANCHERRY, ALMOND AND WHITE CHOCOLATE COOKIES (GF/V)

7 c rolled oats
2 tsp baking soda
1 tsp salt
1 c brown sugar
½ c maple syrup
½ c coconut oil
½ c applesauce
1 mashed banana
4 eggs (I used flax)
1 tsp vanilla
1 c dried cherries and cranberries mixed (I imagine 1 full cup of either would also work)
2 c white chocolate chips (real chocolate chips would also be delightful)
2 c almonds, rough chopped

Preheat oven to 350. Use a food processor or power blender to turn 3 c of the oats into flour. Sift the oat flour together with the baking soda and salt. Combine the sugar, syrup, applesauce, banana, and coconut oil in a bowl and mix until as incorporated as the coconut oil will allow. Add eggs and vanilla and mix until incorporated. At a lower speed (or with a slower hand), add the flour mixture a little at a time. Mix in the remaining oats. Add the fruit, nuts and chips.

Cover the dough and refrigerate it for at least ½ hour. Line or lightly oil baking sheets. Use a spoon or scoop to drop balls of dough onto the baking sheet. Flatten slightly with fork or finger. Bake for about 8 minutes. Rotate pans (and move top to bottom/bottom to top if your oven is like mine). Bake about 8 more minutes or until bottoms are browning and some browning is on top as well – or to your cookie doneness preference. Allow to cool for a few minutes on the baking sheet and remove to wire rack for cooling. Eat, quickly, before the others catch on….. I mean share with loved ones.

EASY PEEZY LEMON SQUEEZY COBBLER OR EP COBBLER (GF)
- this to appease my GF husband's hankering for pie!!

Fruit to cover the bottom of a 9 by 13 pan about 1/2 – 1 inch thick.
2 c oats divided into 1 cup measures
½ c unpacked brown sugar – which translates to about 1/3 packed I'm guessing
¼ c butter
¼ tsp salt (optional – I did not use, but it probably would only improve the flavor)

Pre-heat oven to 350.

Wash and cut if using large fruit and spread in bottom of lightly oiled pan. Mix 1 cup of rolled oats into the fruit and stir around.

In a mixing bowl combine 1 cup oats, butter cut into chunks, brown sugar and salt if using. Mix and mash around until it is small clumps. Spread the small clumps out as evenly as possible over the fruit. Bake for about a half hour, or until lightly browned on top and fruit is fragrant and soft. Serve to pie lovers on pie plates with pie forks and with loving instructions to place, with or without ice cream, in pie hole :-)

GOOD NEIGHBOR CHOCOLATE CHIP COOKIES (V)
- makes enough to share

¾ c coconut oil
½ c applesauce
2 c turbinado or coconut sugar
4 flax eggs (4 Tbs flax meal + 12 Tbs water)
4 tsp vanilla
1 tsp baking soda
½ tsp salt
4 c whole wheat pastry flour

3 c semi-sweet or dark chocolate chip cookies
½ c chopped pecans

Preheat oven to 375. In a medium bowl, combine baking soda, salt, and pastry flour. Set aside. In stand mixer bowl or large bowl, mix together coconut oil, applesauce, and sugar. Beat until thoroughly combined. Add eggs and vanilla and beat until incorporated. Add dry ingredients and continue to mix until it looks like cookie batter. Add mix ins and combine. Drop in cookie sized gobs (I use a cookie batter scoop) onto a greased cookie sheet or one lined with parchment. Bake for 12-15 minutes. Allow to cool for at least 2 minutes on the cookie sheet and then remove to wire racks.

HEALTHY PUMPKIN COOKIES (GF/V)
- adpated from The Joyful Pantry[66]

1 ¼ c pureed pumpkin
¼ c maple syrup
¼ c vegetable oil
1 tsp vanilla
2 1/3 c rolled oats (not instant)
1/3 c brown rice flour
1/3 c that is half brown rice flour and half tapioca flour (or for non-GF, use 2/3 cup whole wheat flour for brown rice and tapioca)
2 tsp cinnamon
½ tsp sea salt
1 tsp baking powder
1/3 c chopped pecans
1/3 c semi-sweet chocolate, chopped (or chocolate chips) or raisins

Preheat the oven to 350 F, with the top rack in the top third of the oven (one position above the middle of the oven). Grease a cookie sheet or use parchment paper. Combine the pureed pumpkin, maple syrup, oil, and vanilla in a large bowl. In a smaller mixing bowl, stir together the oats, flours, cinnamon, salt, and baking powder. Pour the dry ingredients into the wet, mixing just until combined. Stir in the chocolate chips or raisins and nuts. The mixture will not stick together as well as many cookie doughs; do not be alarmed by this. Place heaping tablespoons of dough onto the cookies sheet and bake for 14 to 16 minutes, or until the cookies are lightly golden on the bottom.

INTENSELY GOOD BANANA BREAD (V)

1 c whole wheat flour
½ c all purpose flour
2/3 c regular oats
1 tsp baking soda
1 tsp ground cinnamon

½ tsp salt
½ c brown sugar
¼ c applesauce
2 Tbsp vegetable oil
1/3 c dark molasses
2 large eggs (I used flax)
1 cup mashed ripe banana (about 2 bananas)
¼ c peanut (or other nut) butter
1 tsp vanilla extract
Pecans for the top

Preheat oven to 350°. Combine flours, oats, baking soda, cinnamon, and salt. Place sugar, applesauce, oil, and molasses in a large bowl; beat with a mixer at medium speed until well blended (about 1 minute). Add eggs, banana, nut butter, and vanilla; beat until blended. Add flour mixture; beat at low speed just until moist.

Spoon batter into a greased 8 1/2 x 4 1/2-inch loaf pan. Decorate with pecans. Bake at 350° for 1 hour and 5 minutes or until a wooden pick inserted in center comes out clean. Cool 10 minutes in pan on a wire rack; remove from pan. Eat some while it is warm and the outer crust is at its peak.
Cool completely on wire rack before storing.

MOVIE GORP (GF/V – depending on the granola you use)

5 c popcorn, lightly salted (I don't recommend butter as it will soggify everything)
4 c granola (we have a recipe right here in this book!)
2 c almonds
2 c low sugar cereal
2 c dried fruit

I recommend mixing the granola, almonds, and dried fruit in a large bowl first. Then add the cereal and popcorn and gently mix with your hands. You'll notice that this makes an ENORMOUS amount of GORP, so best prepared for a group, or divided in half. Delish.

MY BEST GF CHOCOLATE CHIP COOKIES (GF/V)
- adapted from I.S. at Yahoo Voices[67]

1 cup Bob's Red Mill GF baking flour
½ c almond meal (or dried and pulverized leftover almond milk mash – that's what I use)
½ c brown rice flour
1 ½ tsp baking powder
1 tsp baking soda

1 Tbsp tapioca starch
1 tsp guar gum
½ c unrefined sugar
½ tsp salt
½ c pure maple syrup
½ Tbsp blackstrap molasses
3 tsp pure vanilla extract
½ cup organic neutral flavored oil (coconut oil works also – changes the flavor)
½ – 2/3 c non-dairy chocolate chips
½ c roughly chopped pecans

Preheat oven to 350°F. Mix the dry except chips and nuts. In a separate bowl, combine the maple syrup, molasses and vanilla, then stir in the oil until well combined. Add the wet mixture to the dry, along with the chips & pecans, and stir until combined. Place ½ Tbsp scoops on a baking sheet lined with parchment paper and flatten a little. Bake for 10 – 12 minutes, rotating halfway through until browning just a tad on the bottom. (If using coconut oil, these will spread out a little – not so with avocado or olive). Cool on a wire rack before removing from tray.As Little Sis always says….. and she comes from a very bright family I hear – Eat that chocolate cookie while it is still warm!!

NECTARINE CREAM PIE WITH WALNUT CRUST (GF/V)

Crust

2 ½ c walnuts
1 tsp baking soda
¼ tsp salt
2 Tbsp coconut oil

Cream Filling

2 c soaked sunflower seeds (soaked in water at least 15 minutes)
½ c coconut milk (or whatever alternative milk you dig)
2 Tbsp maple syrup
1 Tbsp fresh lemon juice
½ tsp vanilla
small handful raw cashews

Super Fab Fruit

2 large ripe nectarines
1 ½ c blueberries
2 Tbsp jam

Preheat oven to 350. Put the ingredients for the crust into food processor bowl and process until nuts are chopped fine. Press into pie pan using a spatula or your fingers. Bake for 30-35 minutes, until the crust browns and is crumbly at the edges. Remove and allow to cool on the counter.

While the crust is baking, put the ingredients for the cream filling into the food processor and process until smooth and creamy, scraping down the sides as necessary. When finished, move to bowl and keep in refrigerator. Slice nectarines and mix blueberries with jam. When the crust has cooled, spread cream filling (I didn't use all of mine and enjoy it on pancakes) into the walnut crust. Be gentle, the crust is delicate. Arrange sliced nectarines however you like and garnish with blueberries. Chill until serving time. Serve modest pieces – it's really satisfying.

NUT BUTTER BLISS BALLS (DF/V Option)
adapted from Diana Herrington's Peanut Butter Bliss Balls[68]

1 c toasted sunflower seeds
1 c nut butter (I have tried almond and peanut, both delicious)
½ c + 1 Tbsp honey or maple syrup
¼ c coconut (unsweetened, flaked)
¼ – ½ c almond flour (can sub coconut flour, which is pricey, or oat flour)
¼ c oats
¼ c raisins
¼ c toasted sesame seeds

Toasting raw sunflower and sesame seeds:
Toast the sunflower seeds at 350 for about 8 minutes – just keep an eye on them so they don't burn, and the sesame seeds for about 5 minutes, again, watch them as ovens are different, pans are different, it's a beautiful variable world!

Variation in flour amount is due to variety of consistency in nut butters. The almond flour we use is the dried out leftovers from making almond milk, so it may be a bit lighter than store bought almond flour – and is definitely cheaper!!

Place toasted sunflower seeds in a bowl with all of the other ingredients except the sesame seeds and smush it all together. Basically you want a dough consistency that is sticky enough to hold together and pick up a coating of sesame seeds but not too sticky to eat. Start with the lowest amount of flour and add more until you like the consistency. Taste tests are totally appropriate and recommended. Pour toasted sesame seeds onto a plate. Form edible size balls (this of course will be affected by the wonderful variety of mouth sizes.… I make mine large) and roll them in the sesame seeds. For more variety you can roll them in unsweetened coconut.

OATY BITES (GF if using GF oats/V)

- makes about 15 bites, unless you'd rather have many small bites or a few big honkin' bites

16 dates
1Tbsp plus 1tsp maple syrup
1Tbsp plus 1tsp water
1tsp vanilla
1/4 c hemp seeds (or whatever nut or seed you prefer)
1.5 c rolled oats, plus a handful for rolling

In a food processor, combine the dates and the liquids. Process until as smooth as you can get it. Add the hemp (I chose hemp because of the nutritional boost and the relative small size to prevent picky kid rejection) and the oats and process until a ball forms and the mixture is sticky but not too terribly wet to the touch. You should be able to form shapes with it. If it seems to sticky, add some more oats. Form into balls and roll in oats.

We prefer ours cool and so keep them in the fridge. There. Voila. Done. No stinkin' icing. No flipping' sprinkles. Just simple ingredients with a sweet touch. Perhaps next time I'll add a little cinnamon and try to shape one like a gorilla.

SPICY SWEETIES (GF/V)
- inspired by oatmeal and chickpea flour cookies on Taste of Beirut[69].

3 ½ c oats
1 c chickpea flour
½ tsp each of salt, baking soda, & baking powder
2 medium bananas (very ripe)
1 egg (I used flax)
¼ c + 1 Tbsp maple syrup
1 tsp + a dash garam masala (or to taste)
1 t vanilla
1/8 c sunflower oil (or other oil)
3 Tbsp tahini (or other nut butter, but the tahini is more delicate than most)
¼ c chocolate chips or chunks or however you like it
¼ c chopped pecans
¼ c shredded unsweetened coconut

Preheat oven to 350. Grind 2 c oatmeal in food processor or heavy duty blender to make oat flour. Add chickpea flour and salt, baking soda, baking powder and pulse to combine. Transfer to bowl and stir in remaining 1 ½ c oats. Combine bananas, egg, maple syrup, garam masala, vanilla, oil and tahini either in bowl of standing mixer or in food processor. (You can, of course also mix these things by hand – I am lazy and have angry finger joints). Add the wet to the dry and mix in whatever way you like to mix cookie dough. When the dough is fully incorporated, add in the mixy bits (chips, nuts and coconut) and stir to combine. Drop onto lined or oiled baking sheet with a scoop or tablespoon. When the pan is full, use a fork or finger to flatten the cookies out. Because there is no butter, they will not melt down the way many butter based cookies do.

Bake for 15-20 minutes until bottoms are brown and there is some browning around the edges. Cool for a couple of minutes on cookie sheet and transfer to wire racks. While they are delicious warm because ANY cookie with chocolate in it is yummy warm, the real fabulous complexity of these babies is best appreciated after cooling, when the garam masala shines through.

SUPER CHOCOLATE PUMPKIN BROWNIES (GF/V)
- adapted from Sarah's awesome Sweet Potato Fudgy Brownies[70]

¼ c coconut oil, melted
2/3 c unsweetened cocoa
1 c rolled oats, blitzed in food processor or blender until flour-like
¼ tsp baking powder
¼ tsp salt
¾ c coconut sugar (or more if you are used to sweeter treats)
2/3 c canned pumpkin
1 flax egg (1 Tbsp flax meal with 3 Tbsp water) or whatever kind of egg works for your tribe
1 ½ tsp vanilla
a couple of handfuls of pecans and chocolate chips (because really, shouldn't you?)

Set oven to 350. Oil a square pan. Combine coconut oil and cocoa in large bowl. Stir until smooth. Combine dry ingredients (except sugar) in small bowl. In another bowl, combine the sugar, pumpkin, flax egg, and vanilla and whisk until the sugar is not so granular. Add chocolate/oil combo. Stir to combine. Add dry ingredients. Stir to combine. Add nuts/chips/whatever floats your brownie boat. Give one last stir and transfer (you will not be pouring) into waiting pan.

Bake for 25 minutes (or so), until the top is dry, maybe even has a crack or two and it feels firm to the touch. If you like 'em drier, leave 'em in longer. Let cool in the pan for a bit, sneak some crispy edges while nobody's looking.

SWEET POTATO COOKIES WITH WALNUTS & DARK CHOC. CHIPS (GF/V)
– based on my very own Crancherry, Almond, and White Chocolate Cookies

3 c almond flour (I made mine from homemade almond milk meal as described in my pal Sarah's post[71], I think you could also use oat flour made by blitzing the mess out of rolled oats as in Crancherry cookies)
2 tsp baking soda
1 tsp salt
½ c preferred solid sweetener (I used turbinado sugar)
½ c maple syrup
½ c coconut oil, melted
1 mashed banana
2/3 c mashed sweet potato
3 eggs (I used flax)
1 tsp vanilla
4 c rolled oats
1 c chopped walnuts (or your preferred nut)
1 c dark chocolate chips

Preheat oven to 350. Sift almond flour with baking soda and salt into small bowl and set aside.
Combine sweeteners, coconut oil, banana, sweet potato in large bowl. Mix to combine (I used a machine for this, although I imagine you could do it by hand. You will want to be sure to be more thorough in mashing your sweet potato in particular.). Add eggs and vanilla to incorporate.
Add small dry bowl to large wet bowl and stir or mix to combine. Stir in oats. Stir in nuts and chocolate. Do NOT drool in the bowl as you do this – it is not socially acceptable, or so I'm told.

Use a tablespoon or scoop to place on parchment lined or greased cookie sheet. Flatten cookies a bit with your finger or a spoon as they will not melt into the traditional cookie shape. Bake for about 18-20 minutes (rotate tray in middle if that's what works for you, and watch the time, my oven is wonky) or until browned to your liking. Cool on baking sheets for a couple of minutes before removing to wire racks to cool. Store in fridge if you have any left.

SWEET POTATO CRUSTED APPLE PIE (GF/V)
crust inspired by – Claire at Just Blither Blather[72]

Crust:
3 c shredded sweet potato
1 tsp coconut oil

1 tsp cinnamon
1 Tbsp maple syrup

Pre-heat oven to 375. Mix together ingredients and press into 9 – 10" pie plate. Bake for 15 minutes.

Filling:

4 apples, chopped into chunks
¼ c oats
¼ c sugar
1 Tbsp cinnamon

Pour filling into crust. Cover loosely with aluminum foil. Bake at 375 for about 35 – 45 minutes. Peek, smell and listen to determine doneness.

ULTIMATE WALNUT CRUST APPLE PIE (GF/DF)
- only slightly changed from: Mark's Daily Apple[73]

2 ½ c walnuts
1 tsp baking soda
¼ tsp kosher salt
2 Tbsp coconut oil, melted (original recipe is same amount of melted butter)

Preheat oven to 350 F. Blend walnuts, baking soda and salt in a food processor until finely ground. Add coconut oil and pulse until oil is mixed in. Scrape the batter into a 9-inch tart pan (I used a standard glass pie plate). You can use a rubber spatula to smooth the batter over the bottom and up the sides, you may need to use your fingers – but the spatula did the job for me. Smooth and pat the batter out evenly. Bake for 15 minutes at 350.

While baking you can assemble this or some other filling:

Apple Crumbly Bumbly Filling:

4 ½ large Fuji or other crisp apples – sliced, chunked, however you like them. The bigger they are the longer they'll take to cook. Just cut enough to make a heap in your pie plate.
½ c granulated sugar
½ c + 1 Tbsp. (or one heaping 1/2 cup) oat flour. (Just whiz some oatmeal in the blender to make oat flour)
1 Tbsp cinnamon

Chop apples. Mix with other ingredients in a bowl and then gently dump into prepared and baked pie crust .The crust will be very soft and puffing up in spots with heat. Dump gently so as not to shove crust away from the plate. Return to oven. Bake for about 20 minutes at 350, then cover with a bit of aluminum foil and bake about another 25 minutes.

Entrees

ANYTHING GOES BURRITOS (GF Option/V Option)

6 Whole grain tortillas / GF tortillas
BEANY FILLING
CHEESY FILLING (vegan version requires soaking first thing in the morning – see cheesy filling section!)
Fresh Veggies

Start with warmed whole-grain tortillas which you can warm at the end according to package directions. Then make fillings that your family can mix and match.

BEANY FILLING:

1 medium onion, finely chopped
1 can beans (I used dark red kidney beans)
several Tbsp water as needed.
dash of oil
¼ – ½ tsp ground cumin
dash of chili powder or to taste
dash of salt

Chop onion and heat oil in a skillet. Add onion and spices & cook several minutes until translucent. Add drained and rinsed beans. Cook on low and mash with a mashing tool of your choice. Add water a bit at a time to give your beany filling a little mush.

This bean dish resembles re-fried beans which is also a fast option, but I found this to be fresher tasting and cheaper, especially if you are using organic beans vs. organic pre-prepared re-fried beans.

CHEESY FILLING:

Option 1: cheese ;-)   Grate some cheese and add it to the burrito assembly line

Option 2: quick sunflower seed / cashew cheese

This is an attempt to combine some cheesy offerings we have shared in the past (sunflower cheese & cashew cheese) but without the extra work and time involved in making firm cashew cheese.

½ c sunflower seeds
½ c cashews
place both in 2 cup measuring cup and add water to the 2 cup line
Place in cup to soak first thing in the morning to be ready for dinner

Baby Steps to Better Health / Recipes: Entrees

juice of ½ lemon (about 2 Tbsp)
½ Tbsp apple cider vinegar
1-2 Tbsp water
2 Tbsp nutritional yeast flakes
1 clove garlic
½ – 1 tsp salt

Mix all in food processor until creamy, scraping down sides as needed

VEGGIES:

Whatever you have that your people will eat, inside of, or next to, a burrito. I had fresh red pepper and romaine. WHATEVER works. Any vegetable is better than no vegetable.

Line it up on the counter or server or dinner table and let everyone make their favorite.

Of course you can use any leftover meat you have as well, but your family will probably not even miss it with the hearty bean and cheese combo. It's a new year and a new horizon…. who knows what they'll try… especially if it's what's on the table ;-)

SLOW COOKER BARLEY, BLACK BEAN and CORN BURRITOS (V)

olive oil for pan
½ c chopped onion
1 clove garlic
1 (15 oz) can black beans (or equivalent dry, soaked and cooked), rinsed and drained
15 oz tomato (diced, crushed, whatever – I used 15 oz leftover homemade pasta sauce)
1 c uncooked pearl barley
1 ½ c water
¾ cup frozen whole-kernel corn
juice of ½ small lime
2 Tbsp Bragg's or soy sauce
1 tsp oregano
1 tsp ground cumin
½ tsp chili powder
½ tsp ground red pepper (opt – I omitted)

Sauté onions for a few minutes and throw the garlic in for a few seconds once the onions are translucent. Transfer to the Crock Pot. Follow with all of the remaining ingredients, stir, put the lid on and cook on low for 4-5 hours. Chop some fresh veggies and cilantro to go with the burritos. Serve with tortillas and cashew, sunflower or whatever you call cheese

(30 MINUTE) BEAN AND BULGUR CHILI (GF/V)

olive oil for the pot/pan
1 onion, chopped
3 large cloves garlic, chopped
3 c lentil/bulgur mixture (in this recipe section)
¼ tsp ground sage
¼ tsp salt
1 green pepper, chopped
1 can drained and rinsed black beans (or 1 ½ c soaked and cooked)
2 large cans diced tomatoes
1 tsp salt
½ tsp chipotle chili powder
1 tsp chili powder
1 tsp oregano

Warm olive oil in skillet over medium. Add lentil bulgur mixture to skillet and LET IT SIT.
You are going for a little browning and crisping here. If you stir too much, you will get neither. Check after you've given it a few minutes, add sage and 1/4 tsp salt to lentil/bulgur, then stir/flip to brown the other sides. Warm olive oil in large pot. Add chopped onions and sauté until onions have softened and become a bit translucent. Add garlic and cook until fragrant. Add green peppers.
When lentil/bulgur mix is browned to your liking, transfer to pot with onions/peppers. Add spices and diced tomatoes. Stir to incorporate. Bring to simmer and let cook to meld flavors, about 15-20 minutes.

BUTTERNUT SQUASH, ONION, POTATO MELEE (GF/V)
- adapted from *The Whole Foods Market Cookbook* "Roasted Butternut Squash with Penne Pasta"

2 medium butternut squash (8 – 10 cups after cubed and peeled)
2 medium diced sweet onions (about 2 cups)
4 cloves minced garlic
¼ – ½ tsp crushed red chili flakes
4 Tbsp olive oil
juice of ½ lemon
2 tsp salt
About 3 c red potatoes cut into chunks
1 ½ c walnuts
1 Tbsp nutritional yeast flakes
freshly ground pepper to taste

Preheat oven to 375. Peel and cube the butternut squash -and yes here is a vegetable that I actually DO peel ;-). Dice those sweet ol' onions and shed a few tears for their goodness

Mince the garlic. Toss the above along with the chili flakes, olive oil, lemon juice and salt in a big bowl and mix. Dump into a baking sheet with sides. Make sure you don't have too much liquid in the bottom of your pan or you won't get good roasting of the garlic or onions, so beware of that as you pour in your melee of orange and white.

Roast for 45 – 60 minutes until desired tenderness, stirring occasionally. While this is roasting, wash and cube your red potatoes and put in a pot of water to boil. Set them boiling about 20 minutes before you expect the squash to be done. It's all right if they are done first and sit in hot water for awhile. 10- 15 minutes prior to squash done-ness, add the 1 ½ c of walnuts and stir around. When done, take out the pan and stir in the nutritional yeast flakes.

CARNI-MOM'S CRABCAKES (DF)
- adapted from the Old Bay Seasoning tin

1 lb. crab meat
8 single saltine crackers (Carni-Mom used gluten free this time – thanks again Mom!)
2 Tbsp. mayonnaise
2 tsp. Old Bay seasoning
chopped fresh parsley (couldn't pin her down on an amount – about a third of a handful was the best we could do)
1/2 tsp. yellow or dijon mustard
1 egg, beaten

Smash crackers into small pieces. Mix in everything but the crab meat. Stir in crab meat. Shape mixture into patties. Broil 6 minutes each side. Eat quickly enough to get seconds, but not so fast that you don't truly savor this wonderful thing.

CASHEW CARROT CURRY (GF/V)
- adapted from *The New Enchanted Broccoli Forest* by Mollie Katzen

4 Tbsp. Coconut Oil (can use Ghee or butter, but I really recommend the coconut oil)
4 crushed garlic cloves
2 tsp freshly grated ginger
2 tsp mustard seeds
2 tsp ground cumin
1 ½ tsp ground coriander
2 tsp dill weed
1 ½ tsp turmeric
2 tsp salt
2 c sliced red onion

4 red potatoes -thinly sliced and don't you dare peel them!! ;-)
6 large carrots – thinly sliced – you may dare, but I wouldn't
2 cups orange juice – I squeezed a couple of oranges, with a little pulp right into the pan
2 red or orange bell peppers, thinly sliced
1 ½ c toasted cashews or pieces
1 c yogurt (I use coconut yogurt)
Cooked brown rice or some other grain to accompany

Melt coconut oil in a large skillet. Add garlic, ginger and mustard seed over medium heat until seeds begin to pop. Add remaining spices and onions. Sauté until translucent. Add potatoes and carrots and cook 5 – 10 minutes. Add orange juice and simmer until potatoes and carrots are almost tender. Add peppers and cook a few more minutes – make sure potatoes are cooked! Turn off heat – mix in yogurt and serve topped with cashews. I do not mix the cashews in during cooking or into leftovers because they become mushy and I prefer them crunchy.

CAULIFLOWER STEAKS with CAPERED TOMATO SAUCE (GF/V)
- adapted from MarthaStewart.com[74]
served 4 with leftovers

3 Tbsp olive oil, divided
3 large cloves garlic, minced, divided
1 large head cauliflower
4 Tbsp capers
1 c diced tomatoes (or leftover tomato sauce)
1 large red pepper
splash red wine vinegar
fresh chopped parsley for garnish

Preheat oven to 400. Wash the cauliflower and remove any remaining leaves. Cut the end of the stem, but be sure to leave the core intact. Cut cauliflower into 1/2 to 3/4 inch slices – slice all the way across the cauliflower. Don't panic if some florets come off – simply set them aside with the small end pieces. Warm 1 Tbsp olive oil in each of 2 pans. Add 1 clove minced garlic into each pan. When oil is warm, add cauliflower. Sprinkle with a little salt. Allow "steaks" to brown (don't fuss with them too much).

When brown (at least, but not likely longer then 4-5 minutes), flip and brown the other side. When both sides are brown, move to baking dish and transfer to oven and roast until tender (12-16 minutes). While the cauliflower roasts, add remaining Tbsp olive oil to one pan. While it warms, chop up the reserved florets/end pieces into small pieces. Roughly chop red pepper. Add the third minced clove of garlic into oil and add cauliflower. Allow to cook for a couple of minutes. Add red pepper & cauliflower, capers and tomatoes and simmer gently until vegetables are tender. Add red wine vinegar when done. Serve cauliflower steak with tomato sauce and fresh parsley. Grin when neither child will eat the sauce. Grin more when they both love it anyway – more sauce for you.

CHICKPEA and CASHEW TIKKA MASALA (GF/V)
– inspired by Vegetarian Times' Chickpea Tikka Masala[75]

olive oil for pan
1 c finely chopped onion
1 ½ Tbsp garam masala
1 ½ Tbsp tomato paste
1 ½ tsp powdered ginger (or 3 t fresh grated – I was out)
½ red or yellow pepper, chopped
2 c cooked chickpeas
3 small cans diced tomatoes
pinch paprika
pinch chipotle or other chile powder to taste
1 c raw cashews
chopped cilantro

Warm oil in large skillet (I used cast iron – the pan should be relatively deep). Add onions and a sprinkle of salt. Sauté onions for about 5 minutes on low-medium heat, until they are translucent. Add tomato paste and spices (other than paprika and chile). Cook for another minute or so – until the spices become fragrant. Add peppers and sauté about another minute. Add chickpeas and tomatoes and bring to a boil. Lower heat to simmer, add cashews and remaining spices. Simmer for at least 15 minutes, stirring occasionally. We served ours with leftover rice and chopped cilantro as a garnish.

CHICKPEA SALAD SAMMIES (GF/V)

2 outer ribs celery, chopped
1/2 red onion (or whatever you like), chopped
2 ½ c cooked or canned (rinsed and drained) chickpeas
4 Tbsp sunflower cheese (or creaminess of your choice)
2 Tbsp dijon mustard
2 Tbsp white wine vinegar
½ – 1 tsp dried thyme
2 tsp dried tarragon
½ t salt
fresh ground pepper to taste
½ avocado, cut into smallish pieces
sprinkle paprika (opt.)
green olives, chopped (opt.)

Combine the chopped celery, onion, and chickpeas in a bowl. In a smaller bowl mix the sunflower cheese, mustard, vinegar, and seasonings. Whisk (or fork it as I usually do) until incorporated. Scrape wet bowl into dry bowl. Stir until they're all playing nicely. Add avocado and stir again to combine. It's okay if the avocado smushes a bit – it will just add to the creaminess of the salad. Serve with a sprinkle of paprika and a dusting of chopped olives. We had ours on whole wheat bread with red lettuce.

CHIPOTLE ROASTED SWEET POTATOES w/ BLACK BEANS AND QUINOA
(GF/V)

1 ½ – 2 pounds sweet potatoes washed (not peeled)
1 generous Tbsp coconut oil, melted if solid
¼ tsp chipotle powder
a couple of shakes garlic powder
a couple of shakes ground cumin
salt to preference
quinoa or rice (enough for your tribe and maybe some leftovers)
cooked black beans (enough for your tribe and maybe some leftovers)
cilantro or parsley garnish (optional)
fresh lime juice garnish (optional)

Preheat oven to 475. While the oven is heating, cut the sweet potatoes into chunks about 1 inch square. Place potatoes in large bowl. Pour on coconut oil and toss to coat. Add spices and seasonings. Toss to disperse. (If you're going to have quinoa too, now would be a good time to start that.) Place on baking sheet lined with parchment or oiled to prevent a catastrophic mess.
Roast for 20-25 minutes, stirring/turning potatoes about halfway through. Serve on a bed of quinoa (or rice) with some black beans and toppings if desired.

CINNAMON CABBAGE STIR FRY (GF/V)

3/4 head of a cabbage chopped small (about 6 c)
2 – 3 carrots chopped (about 1 c)
1 large yellow or red pepper, chopped
1 – 2 Tbsp coconut oil
1 Tbsp cumin seed
1 Tbsp cinnamon
1/2 onion – chopped
1 large clove garlic
1 tsp salt
1/2 c water to help steam the cabbage
raisins for garnish

hot sauce (to personal taste – right on each helping!
Whatever you would like to serve this over.

I chose to serve this over yellow lentils which are a mild and soft lentil that cooks quickly and provides more protein than using rice. But you are free to use rice or some other grain!

1 cup yellow lentils
2.5 cups water

Combine lentils and water and set on high until boiling. Then cover and simmer on low for about 25 minutes or until soft.

While the lentils are cooking:
Chop vegetables. Heat coconut oil on medium in large pan or pot. Add cumin seed, cinnamon, and salt. Heat until seeds start to pop then add carrots and peppers for a few minutes. Add cabbage and cover, stirring frequently and turning down to avoid burning. After 5 minutes, add 1/2 cup water and re-cover to help steam the cabbage. Cook until desired tenderness. Drain lentils if too soupy. Serve over lentils or grain and garnish with raisins and a touch of hot sauce to personal taste.

COCONUT CURRY WITH GREEN BEANS, POTATOES & KALE (GF/V)
- adapted from Ron Mikulac's Green Beans, Potatoes & Spinach in Coconut Curry[76]

2 Tbsp coconut oil (or vegetable oil)
1 ½ tsp salt
1 tsp turmeric
1 Tbsp brown mustard seeds
½ tsp garam masala
1 tsp cayenne (optional)
large can or box diced tomatoes
1 c water
about 5 medium russet potatoes, washed and cut into 1 inch pieces
3 large handfuls green beans trimmed (cut if you like, I didn't)
1 ½ c coconut milk (the full fat canned kind)
3 VERY large handfuls baby or cut kale

In deep pan or large pot, melt coconut oil. Add spices and stir a bit. Sauté until mustard seeds begin to pop and your kitchen smells AH-MAZING. Add tomatoes and stir. Allow to warm, stirring a few times. Add 1 c water and potatoes. Stir. Allow to come to a gentle boil, cover and turn down to simmer for about 10 minutes. Stir occasionally ensuring potatoes aren't sticking to the bottom.

Add the green beans and continue to cook for about 4 more minutes or until the beans and potatoes are tender to your liking, stirring occasionally. Add the coconut milk and warm. (If coconut milk is pasty you can throw it in the blender first making it blend in the curry better and it will be a prettier dish, but you don't have to) Add the kale and stir. Cook just until the kale wilts (gets softer, but not mushy). Serve on top of rice – or your preferred grain.

COLD SESAME NOODLES (V)

1 lb noodles (I used 100% whole wheat, but it's your call)
¼ sesame oil
3 Tbsp Bragg's liquid aminos or Soy Sauce
2 Tbsp rice wine vinegar (I used brown)
2 Tbsp tahini
2 Tbsp peanut butter
1 Tbsp maple syrup (or sweetener of your choice)
2 ½ tsp chili garlic paste
2 tsp sesame seeds (toast if you like, I didn't)
2 cloves minced garlic
2 spring onions, sliced (opt.)
1 tsp finely chopped ginger
2 carrots, julienned
1 cucumber julienned
other veggies as available and desired i.e. peas, spinach, sprouts, roasted broccoli

Cook the noodles – be sure you have a BIG pot. Inferior noodle results are often a result of crowding the pot – too many noodles, not enough water. Goodness knows you don't want inferior noodle results. When cooked to your liking, drain noodles, place sesame oil in large bowl and add noodles. This step can be done ahead of time. I let mine sit this way for a few hours with no problem. Put all the other ingredients except the veggies into a bowl, food processor or blender and mix. Pour over cooled noodles. Add veggies and stir OR serve noodles, veggies and sesame seeds for garnish at the table so individual munchers can find their own perfect cucumber/noodle/carrot ratio.

COOL STIR FRY SALAD (GF/V)

2 ½ cups dry rice, cooked to package directions, or your usual way! (I like brown basmati)
¼ head cabbage, shredded

~~~~~~~~~~ar

r, grated

stems from 3 large beets

3 carrots, sliced into coins
2 cups broccoli florets
3 – 5 Tbsp Bragg's liquid amino acids (or soy sauce) – I used 4
½ – 1 ½ Tbsp sesame oil - I used 1
1 cup roasted almonds (or raw)

Prepare rice according to package directions (For added flavor cook rice in broth, stock or a mix of broth and water). When done, set aside to cool. Place cabbage in a large bowl and add rice vinegar and 1 tsp sesame oil. Stir and leave to sit. Almonds can be roasted in a 375 oven for 10 minutes laid out flat if you want to roast them. Chop and sauté garlic, ginger, beet stems and greens. Start with garlic and sauté for a few minutes, add ginger for another minute then the chopped stems for about 3 or 4 minutes and finally the greens to wilt. Set aside to cool.

Chop the rest of the veggies and cook or leave raw as you prefer. I just barely cooked my broccoli florets, but not necessary. Mix everything but the Bragg's and extra sesame oil in the large bowl with the cabbage and stir. Add the Bragg's (or soy sauce) and sesame oil a bit at a time, stir and taste. Extra vinegar can be added at this point as well if you like. Serve at room temperature or chilled – we've enjoyed it both ways

CREAMED KALE DINNER (GF/V)

This can be made as a side dish or by mixing in some rice or quinoa, a heartier dish. I love to keep leftover cooked rice and/or quinoa in the fridge for these types of quick and easy meals.

If using grain – cook enough ahead of time that it will be done!
kale – broken into pieces and de-stemmed, enough to stuff a 4 cup measuring cup.

Vegan Cream Sauce:

¼ c finely chopped onion
1 clove minced garlic
½ c soaked cashews (at least 6 hours in twice as much water)
4 Tbsp nutritional yeast flakes
1 ½ – 2 Tbsp prepared mustard
1 tsp salt
2 tsp lemon juice
1 c non-dairy, unsweetened milk
1 small squirt honey (probably ½ tsp)
1 Tbsp flour (I used brown rice)

Sauté the onion and garlic in a little olive oil. Meanwhile place all other ingredients except kale in a food processor. When onion and garlic is translucent add to the food

Baby Steps to Better Health / Recipes: Entrees 170.

processor. Process baby. Processing is so very good! Add the kale to the pan you sautéed the onion and garlic in – add 2 Tbsp of water, stir, cover and steam. Once the kale gets a bit wilty add your sauce. Cook just a couple of minutes to warm and mix. Then add a cup or two of rice or quinoa or some other grain. If you are not going to mix in grain you might want to either cut the sauce in half – or save some for another use the next night.

EASIEST ZUCCHINI 'GNA' (GF Option/V) (as in the last syllable of lasagna – pronounced nyah!)

2 zucchini – sliced
1 package tofurky Italian sausage (14 oz.) or your fave
about 1/3 box crackers (I used GF crackers)
oil for baking dish (used coconut oil)
1 tsp each of oregano & thyme if not using seasoned sausage
salt to taste

Preheat oven to 350. Oil covered baking dish. Place layer of zucchini (a couple of slices thick) on the bottom and alternately layer other items until done. Bake, covered, for about 20 minutes or until tender.

EGGPLANT ROLLATINI (GF/V)

1 medium sized eggplant
1 c cheese type (or cheeze type in this case) filling
herbed olive oil for drizzle
fresh tomatoes (or leftover tomato sauce) for condiment

Cheeze Filling

1 c sunflower cheez (in our appetizers and dippers section – leave out the dill)
1 c moxerella[77] cheese (vegan mozzarella cheese – recipe link below)

Put in food processor. Blitz. Done.

Herbed Olive Oil

½ c olive oil
small handful basil

I put these into a blender and made lovely green herby oil, but there's no reason you couldn't chop the basil and add it to the oil by hand.

Cut the eggplant into slices 1/3 inch or less (or they'll be unrollable). Sprinkle slices with salt and let stand (to remove some moisture). Rinse the slices and blot dry. Brown in a warm pan with oil. Remove from heat. When cool enough to manage, plop about 2 Tbs of filling in the center and roll it up – secure with toothpick if necessary. These can be stored in a baking dish, in a single layer covered with foil until you are ready to eat (i.e. great make-ahead dish). When ready, preheat oven to 400 and bake until warm through 20-25 minutes. Serve with herbed olive oil and tomatoes (or sauce).

GINGERED MUSHROOMS, GREENS & CARROTS with BLACK RICE (GF/V)

¼ c mirin
2 tsp Bragg's, tamari or soy sauce
1 Tbsp rice vinegar
2 Tbsp corn starch
olive oil for the pan
1 lb mushrooms, sliced thickly
2 carrots, sliced
2 Tbsp fresh ginger, minced or grated
3 cloves garlic, chopped
6-8 large handfuls of tender greens
½ c veggie broth
4 c cooked black rice (or brown rice, soba noodles, whatever you prefer)
2 Tbsp sesame seeds

Stir the first four ingredients in a small bowl and set aside. Warm a skillet and add a very small amount of olive oil to warm. Place mushrooms in the pan and allow to cook for a few minutes, stirring occasionally. Mushrooms will release water as they cook. Add carrots, ginger and garlic and cook for another minute or two. Add broth and mirin mixture, and continue to cook for several minutes while the liquid reduces and thickens, stirring occasionally. Add greens at the last possible minute to prevent them from becoming overcooked - bright green and just wilted.
Serve over whatever grain or starch you've got going.

GLUTEN FREE FRANKENPATTIES (GF/V)

½ onion chopped
1 large clove garlic, smashed
1 ¼ c chickpeas (I suspect any bean would work)
¾ c almond milk mash (leftover from making almond milk, alternatively I would suggest using mashed potatoes)
2 oz kale (a couple of generous handfuls, any hearty green would work)
2 Tbsp sunflower cheese (or mayo)
3 Tbsp almond milk (or other liquid)
2 Tbsp tahini (or other nut butter)
1 ½ Tbsp Bragg's or soy sauce

1 tsp salt
¾ tsp dry yellow mustard
2/3 c garbanzo flour (you could probably use just about any flour here, although I like the flavor, and the gluten free-ness of the chickpea)
1 ½ c cooked quinoa (or rice or whatever other grain you have leftover)

Preheat oven to 325. Warm pan on stove with a splash of olive oil. Add onions and cook on low-medium until onions are soft. Add garlic and cook until you can smell it (about 30 seconds). Put contents of pan and other ingredients except garbanzo flour and quinoa into a food processor. You may need to add the kale a little at a time. Add the flour a bit at a time until the mixture is wet, but will hold shape. In a bowl, add the quinoa and stir to distribute. Form dough into patties. If the mixture is too wet, add bit more flour. Add olive oil to pan and warm over medium heat.
Cook patties about 6-8 minutes per side and then move to oven for about 10 minutes to cook through. Yummy with your favorite burger fixins or with a nice big dollop of smoky baba ghanoush.

HEALTHY BECHAMEL WITH KALE AND MUSHROOMS (GF/V)
- sauce from a recipe for mushroom lasagna with garlic-tofu sauce by Kathy Hester in *The Vegan Slow Cooker*, (p. 106)

Sauce:
1 package silken or soft tofu
Juice of ½ lemon
1 c water
3 cloves garlic or 1 tsp dried
½ to 1 tsp salt
1 ½ Tbsp bouillion (I use Edward and Sons veggie bouillion)
¼ c nutritional yeast flakes

The rest (my adaptation)

1 lb. mushrooms of your choice
1 large bunch greens of kale or other hearty green
Noodles or grain of your choice prepared according to package directions

Purée all the sauce ingredients in a blender and blend until smooth. Sautée sliced mushrooms in a bit of oil of your choice until smaller and more tender. Add as much kale as you can fit in the pan and still stir a bit and get a lid on. Put it in right on top of the mushrooms as the juice from your mushrooms is going to help steam the kale. Stir so it's all wet and put the lid on. Stir a few times until it's looking a bit limp. Add sauce and stir so all is heated. Serve over grain or noodle of your choice

HERBED CHICKPEA SALAD (GF/V)

2 c cooked chickpeas
2 tsp olive oil
juice of about ½ small lemon
2 tsp dried rosemary
½ tsp salt
2 Tbsp chopped celery leaves (or parsley)
ground black pepper to taste

Throw in bowl, toss, done.

HERBED ZUCCHINI RICE (GF/V)

3 medium zucchini, grated (no seeds)*
olive oil for pan
1 onion, chopped as fine as you prefer
2 cloves of garlic, crushed or minced
4 c cooked grains (I mixed quinoa and rice)
1-2 tsp dried tarragon (or herb or your choice)
salt to taste
dash pepper
juice of ½ medium lemon
½ c sunflower cheese (or soft dairy cheese like ricotta)
chopped parsley (optional)

* For this dinner I grated the zucchini. It is important to grate only the skin and the flesh, not the core and seeds of the zuke as the "interior" of the squash contains a lot of water and has a less pleasant texture when cooked, in my opinion. The short version is to grate it down to the core, place in a strainer with a little salt and let it rest for at least 10 minutes.

While the zucchini is resting, warm the oil in a pan. Chop the onion, add to the pan and let cook on med-low heat until translucent. Return to the zucchini and press as much water out as you can with a spoon or squeeze in a towel (over the sink). Add garlic to onion in pan and cook until fragrant. Add zucchini to pan and sauté for about 5 minutes. Add tarragon (you could use another herb, but the tarragon gave a nice fresh and light taste), salt, and pepper. Add rice (or whatever) and sunflower cheese (or whatever) to pan and lower heat – you're warming, not frying. Stir occasionally. When warm, add lemon juice and stir through. We served ours with chopped parsley on top. Easy, soopah fast, and delish!

INSTANTLY HEALTHIER MAC & CHEESE

adapted from Instant mac & cheese recipe on Cooks.com

Sauce:
1 cup cold milk
2 Tbsp White whole wheat flour (what I used)
½ – ¾ tsp salt
¼ tsp dry mustard
¼ – ½ tsp pepper
2 Tbsp Butter
¾ cup grated cheddar cheese (Little Sis' kids preferred less cheese, and they are awfully cute as well… Just sayin')

Set water on to boil for pasta (preferably whole grain)*.

Make the sauce:

Mix the flour and milk in a small jar with a tight-fitting lid. Shake well to mix the flour in. Begin the butter melting in a saucepan over medium high heat. Add the spices and milk/flour mixture making sure to give another good shake to the jar before pouring the milk in. Heat the mixture to boiling, stirring well. Boil, stirring the whole time for 1 minute. Turn heat to low and add cheese. Mix well. Pour over cooked pasta You can freeze some of the sauce for another quick macaroni meal that a kid can easily prepare.

*I am a dumper not a measurer of things like pasta so I'm afraid I don't have a set amount of pasta for this recipe – but leftover sauce can be frozen, and leftover pasta can be saved, so please forgive the lapse. Plus you can find your optimal amount of sauce per bowl of pasta when unencumbered by rigid amounts. Good justification for not having to make this recipe right this second, don't you think? Even though it wouldn't take long at all.

LEFTOVERLICIOUS LENTIL CASSEROLE (GF/V Option) (I always double this).

3c veggie or chicken broth
3/4c lentils
1/2c brown rice
3/4c chopped fresh onion
1/2tsp sweet Basil
1/4tsp oregano
1/4tsp thyme
1 clove garlic, mashed
1/2c shredded cheese (Completely Optional)

I have found the Crock Pot to be the best method for this casserole. Place all ingredients in crock. Cook on low for 2 hours, high for 2 hours. If you are using cheese, spread it on the top of the casserole for the last 25 minutes of cooking. I assume you could simply leave it on low for longer, but I usually need it to be done sooner rather than later. So there you are, a hands-off Sunday dinner that will make leftover lunch too!

LEMON ORZO WITH SPINACH AND ASPARAGUS (V Option)

1 lb. whole wheat orzo
About 5 very large and packed handfuls of raw spinach (adjust to taste)
Juice from 1.5 small lemons
3 T olive oil
2T oregano
salt and pepper to taste
Chopped raw asparagus bits (we used three stalks, but more would have been nicer)
Grated parmesan, if desired

Cook orzo according to package directions – with the caveat that I usually shave a minute or so off of their recommended time. Taste it early, see what you think. You do NOT want a big bowl of mush. While orzo is cooking, chop the spinach into bite sized pieces. Place spinach, lemon juice, and olive oil in large bowl. When orzo is done, drain in sieve or other colander with SMALL holes (sorry if that's obvious, but I've done such things). Add hot orzo to bowl with spinach, etc. and stir, distributing the spinach and seasonings throughout the orzo. Add salt and pepper to taste. Sprinkle asparagus over individual servings. Garnish with parmesan if desired. I went without and didn't miss it. This recipe made plenty for our family of four (with only one reluctant participator – our picky girl, who wasn't even swayed by the promise of stinky pee later) and also served as a leftover dinner for a very hungry adult a couple of nights later.

A Note on Preparing Asparagus: Store-bought asparagus can be tough at the base of the stalk. Test your asparagus by bending one stalk to see how low you can break it easily. Use this stalk as a guide for chopping the bottoms off the rest. If the stalks are particularly thick or seem slightly tough generally, you can also use a vegetable peeler to remove the outer skin, revealing the yummy tender inside.

LENTIL APPLE WALNUT LOAF (GF/V)
- adapted from Angela Liddon[78]

1 cup uncooked lentils
1 cup walnuts, chopped and toasted
3 tbsp ground flax + 1/2 cup water
3 garlic cloves, minced

1 ½ c diced sweet onion
1 c diced celery
1 c grated carrot
½ c peeled and grated sweet apple (use a firm variety)
1/3 cup raisins
½ c rice flour or other gluten free flour
¾ c rolled oats
1 tsp dried thyme
salt & pepper, to taste (I use about 3/4 tsp

Balsamic Apple Glaze:

¼ c ketchup
1 Tbsp pure maple syrup
2 Tbsp apple butter (or unsweetened applesauce in a pinch)
2 Tbsp balsamic vinegar

Preheat oven to 325. Rinse, strain and pick over lentils in case of small rocks. Place lentils into pot along with 3 cups of water (or veg broth). Bring to a boil and season with salt. Reduce heat to medium/low and simmer, uncovered, for at least 40-45 minutes. Stir frequently & add touch of water if needed. Over-cook the lentils slightly so they are very soft. Mash lentils slightly with a spoon when ready. Toast walnuts at 325F for about 8-10 minutes. Set aside.

Increase oven temp to 350. (mine toasted longer because I forgot to set the timer and they were fine ;-). Whisk ground flax with water in a small bowl and set aside. Heat a teaspoon of olive oil in a skillet over medium heat. Sautée the garlic and onion for about 5 minutes. Season with salt.
Add in the diced celery, shredded carrot, apple. Sautée for about 5 minutes more. Remove from heat. Add raisins.

In a large mixing bowl, mix all ingredients together. Adjust seasonings to taste. Grease a loaf pan (or 2 depending on size of your loaf pan. I doubled this and got three 7½"x3½" pans full). Press mixture firmly into pan. While cooking, whisk glaze ingredients. Bake for 40-50 minutes, uncovered. Edges will be lightly brown. Cool for at least 10 minutes before serving. Put some sauce on top ☺ Angela Liddon uses half of the glaze during the baking.

LENTIL BULGUR MIXTURE (V) (meat substitute used in several following recipes)
- from The Tightwad Gazette***

4c water
1c lentils (I used plain brown, super cheap, lentils)
1c bulgur (a form of wheat – health food store / some grocery stores will have it)

Bring water to a boil, add lentils and bulgur and simmer for 45 minutes. Do check and stir periodically as they will stick on the bottom, particularly if you over cook. When finished, turn off heat, leave cover on and let them steam a bit to make the bottom sticking phenomenon go away (works with rice too, by the way). I doubled this recipe and we now have far more of this mixture than we can use in a reasonable amount of time. I will try freezing, but remember that this is an expandy food when you make your own. This mixture should be refrigerated once cooked. Feel free to make the mixture ahead of time by a few days and save yourself some meal prep time

LENTIL BULGUR BURGERS (V option) (say that 10 times fast!)
- adapted from The Tightwad Gazette***

2 c lentil-bulgur mixture
2 c bread crumbs
1 c chopped onion
1/2 c chopped green pepper (optional)
4 T mixed herbs (I use basil, oregano and thyme)
4 cloves garlic
2 eggs (flax, soy, or chicken)
2 T soy sauce or Bragg's plus milk to make 1/2 c (I used almond)
1/4 c sunflower seeds (optional, but I like the texture)

Preheat oven to 350 if you want to bake your burgers. Mix the first six ingredients. Add eggs and soy sauce/milk and mix well. Stir in sunflower seeds.

If you have time, chill your burger mix for at least half an hour (I did it without the chill and it wasn't a big problem). Form into patties. Fry 10 minutes per side, or bake (on parchment or lightly greased cookie sheet) at 350 ten minutes per side. The fried version has a more burger-like appearance, so if you're looking to convince someone, that may be a better approach. I find baking easier in process and for cleanup.

Baby Steps to Better Health / Recipes: Entrees

LUSCIOUS LAYERS (GF/V Option)
- this is a use up what's in your veggie bin kind of recipe, although zucchini does make a nice easy layer… but not necessary.

Corn tortillas (about 1 – 12 for a 9X13 casserole dish)
about 6 cups of sliced veggies (preferably sliced the long way if possible)
I suggest zucchini, tomatoes, yellow squash, spinach
1 onion
mozzarella cheese (or other melty cheese you like) or vegan cheese
either salsa or seasoned tomato sauce

Preheat oven to 350. Lightly oil a baking dish. Sauté the onion adding 2-3 tsp. seasonings that are appropriate to your sauce:
> tomato sauce? Add oregano, basil, rosemary, and/or thyme
> salsa? Add cumin, oregano, coriander, and/or chili powder

If using greens like spinach or swiss chard, add to the pan when onion is translucent and cook til wilted. Place a layer of corn tortillas on the bottom of the pan. Then layer zucchini or squash thinly sliced longways. Layer of cheese and then sauce or salsa. Layer of sautéed onions and greens and more veggies and…Repeat layers as you like.

Bake at 350 for 30 – 45 minutes until zucchini is soft as you like

MINI NEATLOAVES (V Option)
served our family of 4 two dinners with 2 adult lunches left
- Inspired by Confetti Mini-Meatloaf on Spark Recipes

4c lentil-bulgur mix (recipe in this section)
3c rolled oats
1 med onion
2 garlic cloves
2/3c mushrooms (I used reconstituted dried)
2/3 c diced tomatoes (or tomato sauce – we had leftover pasta sauce to use up)
1 small zucchini
2 medium carrots
2 eggs (I used flax eggs)
1 t mustard powder
2 t marjoram
1T creaminess (milk, mayo, yogurt)
3T Braggs liquid aminos or soy sauce

Preheat oven to 350. Lightly oil two muffin tins – you can also use a loaf pan, but I'm just gonna tell you that's not as fun. If you're making flax eggs, prepare them first so they have time to set up. Put lentil-bulgur mix and oats in large bowl. Put veggies in food processor and process until they are no longer distinguishable as individual bits to your pickiest eater (you may not need to be quite as thorough as I was on this front). Add veggie slush to bowl. Add spices and flax eggs and mix. I added about of cup of leftover peas that were in my fridge. (My two still love measuring so they helped a lot on this part). Mix until well combined.

Recruit volunteers to fill muffin tins with neat loaf mix. Bake in oven for about 25-30 minutes (Watch closely as we had little people crises and I'm not sure I got the time exactly right.) If you make a loaf, you will need to cook it longer. If you make one enormous meatball, you'd better make a lot of spaghetti.

MUNG BEAN STEW (GF/V)
- minimally adjusted from Mung Bean Stew on a Budget on Green Kitchen Stories[79]

2 c dried mung beans, soaked in clean water for at least 8 hours
olive oil for the pan
1 medium onion, chopped small
4 cloves garlic, chopped small
1 tsp cumin
6 c water
1 tsp salt
1 can full fat coconut milk
at least 3 c cooked rice (I used brown jasmine and the flavor really complimented the stew)
5 large handfuls fresh spinach (I imagine other greens would work here)

If you need to make rice fresh, start the rice first. Warm olive oil on medium-low in a pan and add the onions. Sprinkle with a small amount of salt and allow the onions to cook for several minutes (at least 5), stirring occasionally to prevent sticking. When onions are softened and translucent, add garlic and cumin and cook until fragrant (30 seconds to a minute). Add water, salt and the mung beans and bring to a boil. Cover and lower heat, simmering for about 30 minutes. Taste to see if bean softness meets your liking. If the greens you're using is of a less tender variety (like kale), add it now and cook for a few minutes to wilt in the soup, then add coconut milk, remove from heat, and stir. If you're using a tender green (like baby spinach), add the coconut milk first, keeping soup on very low heat, add greens, stir and cook for just another minute to help wilt greens. Serve over warm rice.

MUSHROOMS PIGNOLI (GF/V)

Cooked short grain brown rice
Cremini mushrooms, sliced thick
Olive oil and salt for pan
pine nuts

fresh basil, cut (not minced)
lemon wedges (optional)

I've left out measurements because, as is our tradition, we left it all separate and combined it at the table, allowing each person to adjust the ratio of individual components to their own liking.

Warm olive oil in pan over medium heat. Add mushrooms and sprinkle salt over them. Let them alone for long enough to get a little caramelization (some browning that is yummy – if you move them too much, they will not brown, but will still taste very good). Flip the mushrooms over to let the other side brown a little, but take them off the heat while they still have some moisture left in them – don't let them dry out. Serve mushrooms over rice, with pine nuts (you could toast these for more yum), a sprinkle of basil and some lemon if you like.

MUSTARD TEMPEH (GF/V)

This is one of my fave old recipes and one of the first that I could truly claim as my own – not that it's dazzlingly brilliant or anything – just not based heavily on another recipe. I stopped making it because it seems like the price of tempeh went way up, so it is now a bit of a luxury. How does a hunk of fermented soybean cake get to be so expensive? Well, I've never made it, so I guess I can't answer that. But it is good for you and so I indulged… and my son approved it for THAS (thermos @ school). Big thumbs up.

Oil for sauté
1 med – large onion, chopped
2 Tbsp mustard seeds
1/2 Tbsp ground cumin – or more if you have seed which is better
salt to taste – start with ½ tsp.
2 -8oz cakes of tempeh
2 Tbsp dijon mustard
3 Tbsp applesauce
1/8 – 1/4 cup water
Whole grain to serve under or beside

Prepare whole grain according to package directions. Heat some oil in a pan on medium heat and add mustard seed and cumin until seeds begin to pop. Draw pictures in the seeds with your spatula or read your partners fortune in the seeds…. "You have an awesome partner who is cooking this nice meal for you." Add the onion and some salt and cook until onions are becoming translucent. Chop your tempeh into bite sized-ish pieces. Add tempeh to the mix and allow to brown a little / get glistening. Add dijon and applesauce. Add water a bit at a time to achieve a little sauciness… but don't go so far as to make it cheeky or disrespectful ;-). Serve it over (or beside) your grain of choice.

MY FIRST NAMUL (GF/V)

serves 2 as the main event, 4 as a side

4 c spinach, washed and dried
2 t soy sauce (or Bragg's)
2 t toasted sesame oil
1 small clove garlic, made small however you like
1 t sesame seeds

Place everything but sesame seeds in large bowl and toss. Ideally you should massage this with your hands. I was doing a bunch of other things at the same time, and decided to use utensils instead. Set aside and let marinate for 20-30 minutes, tossing periodically. Add sesame seeds, toss and serve. Yes, that's it. How to eat it? You could use it as a side dish for any protein you like. OR you could do what I did and serve it on top of brown rice with warmed frozen peas and a chopped up asparagus stalk. Delish.

NOFREDO ORZO w/ CHICKPEAS, PEAS AND KALE (V)

The Pasta

1 lb whole wheat orzo (can substitute a grain here)
1 c chickpeas
1 c peas (I used warmed frozen)
chopped fresh basil

The Sauce

1 c pine nuts
2 Tbsp olive oil
2 Tbsp nutritional yeast flakes (opt.)
1 Tbsp white wine vinegar
¼ c water
1 tsp salt
1 c steamed cauliflower pieces
fresh ground pepper

Put the water on to boil for pasta. Put all sauce ingredients but pepper into a food processor and process until smooth. Add pepper to taste. When pasta (grain) is done, add chickpeas and peas to the pasta and then add the amount of nofredo your tribe will go for. Serve over a bed of chopped fresh kale. Garnish with chopped basil. I used about half of the sauce to make the dish and then brought the rest to the table so we could add to individual servings as desired.

NUTSHROOM BURGERS (GF/V) or Meatballs!!*

½ c onion
1 clove garlic
2 c cooked leftover grain (I used quinoa)
½ c black beans (I imagine other soft beans would work)
¼ c peanut butter
½ c walnuts
1 c rough cut mushroom
2 Tbsp Bragg's or soy sauce
½ tsp dried rosemary (yes, really)
1 c finely chopped mushroom (I used portobello, but to each his own mushroom)
1 c rolled oats
½ c flaxmeal

Throw the first 9 ingredients into a food processor and process until smooth-ish and well incorporated. I chose to add my walnuts late to retain a little texture. Spoon batter into a large bowl and add the remaining three ingredients. Stir to incorporate. Fashion into patties of whatever shape and size floats your burger boat. I happened to reach this point relatively early in my day, so refrigerated the patties at this point for about 45 minutes with no ill effect.
When you are 20 minutes from dinner, heat a small amount of oil (I used olive oil) in a pan. Cook burgers for a total of 15 minutes or so, flipping as needed to prevent burning.
This recipe made dinner for four and two leftover lunches for two enthusiastic grownups.

* For meatballs: roll the mixture into balls instead of patties – prepare in the frying pan, allowing to sit and brown on as many sides as possible and then place in a baking dish and heat at 325 in the oven for about 20 minutes.

PAKISTANI LENTIL KIMA (GF/V)
– adapted from *More with Less* by Doris Janzen Longacre

3 Tbsp coconut oil
1 c chopped onion
1 clove of garlic, minced
2 potatoes, rough cut 1 inch pieces
1 Tbsp curry powder
1 ½ tsp salt
dash pepper

dash each cinnamon, ginger, and turmeric
2 ½ c diced tomatoes
2 c fresh green beans, cut in half
2 c cooked lentils

Warm coconut oil in pan. Sauté onions on med heat until they are a little translucent. Add garlic and stir until fragrant. Add potatoes and stir to coat with coconut oil. Add spices and stir to coat. Let cook for a minute or so. Add tomatoes. Turn heat down to simmer and cover. Cook about 15 minutes; check potatoes for doneness and simmer until nearly cooked through. Add green beans and cover. Simmer for an additional 5 minutes (more or less to your green bean doneness preference). Add lentils and stir. Heat until lentils are warm. Serve over rice (or whatever grain you have on hand). We garnished with a little coconut and fresh cilantro.

PAN ROASTED POTATOES WITH CHICKPEAS AND GREENS (GF/V)

olive oil for the pan
one onion, sliced
fresh potatoes (enough to feed your crew), sliced as thin as you can manage
salt, pepper to taste
½ tsp oregano
1 ½ c chickpeas (soaked and cooked or if canned – drained and rinsed)
large bunch of greens of your choosing

Preheat oven to 375. Warm olive oil over medium heat in oven safe pan. Sauté onions with a little salt to carmelize (turn brown, not black). Add potatoes to pan with a bit of salt.
Let them be so potatoes can begin to brown. When browning, stir potatoes to brown other side.
Add oregano and pepper. Remove potatoes/onions from stove and place in hot oven for about 15 mins (or until fork tender – will depend on how thin they are cut). Return to stove top. Add chickpeas and stir. Add handfuls of greens and stir. Cook only until greens are wilted.

PANTRY POT PIE (V Option)

The basic idea here is to make a crust and turn leftovers into a pot pie. This can be vegan or not – it all depends on how you make your crust and what you put inside!

We'll start with a vegan crust (what the heck –try it, it's easy!)

EASY VEGAN SAVORY PIE CRUST
- adapted from Little House in the Suburbs' Perfect Pie Crust[80]

2 ¼ c whole wheat pastry flour – spoon measured (not scooped directly out of bag or container)
1 tsp salt
½ c olive oil
¼ c alt milk (I used unsweetened coconut)

Preheat oven to 350. Grease the container you plan to use for your pot pie (loaf pan, deep casserole dish, deep pie plate….) Place flour and salt into a mixing bowl and stir to combine.

Measure out olive oil and milk (use the same container, but don't mix them). Pour the liquid into the dry and stir to combine. I usually ditch the spoon and work with my hands once the flour is mostly incorporated. Knead a little to be sure flour is absorbed. Roll out dough as per the containers you're using, rolling in a pattern so that you're not just rolling in one direction.

I go top to bottom, left to right, diagonal, diagonal until it's about 1/8th inch thick.

Then you can fill your greased dish with some of our suggested leftover combinations or whatever is in your fridge! Place your crust on top – pinch it around the edges. Brush with olive oil if it looks dry. Bake for about 40 minutes or until some bubbling up of filling is starting to happen and the dges are browning.

Here are our suggestions for fillings:

Pantry Pot Pie:

leftover lentil rice casserole
leftover peas
2/3 c shredded cheese (vegan or not)

Place casserole on the bottom, then peas, then cheeses

Mexican Pot Pie:

<u>Slow Cooker Burrito Filling</u>
Diced Tomatoes
Cheese (vegan or not)

Veggie Barley Pot Pie:

<u>Slow Cooker Veggie, Bean, Barley Stew</u>
Fresh Parsley
Cheese (vegan or not)

Walnut Apple Pot Pie:

Baby Steps to Better Health / Recipes: Entrees

<u>Waldorf Sauté</u>
Fresh finely chopped celery
Cheese (vegan or not)

<u>(PICADILLO</u> (GF/V Option)
(Adapted from a recipe given me by my Sis-in-law, from a friend of hers – tried to find it online and couldn't find this one)

1 & 1/2 lbs. ground turkey

OR

3/4 cup lentils cooked in 2 cups of broth. Boil water, add lentils, lower heat, simmer until soft. Add a little more water if it disappears entirely, but don't leave it soupy in the end.

1 Tbsp olive oil
2 cloves crushed garlic
1 large onion, chopped
1 large bell pepper of any color
1 15 oz. can diced tomatoes undrained – or about 1 ½ c diced tomatoes if you have fresh.
6 oz. can tomato paste
½ cup dry sherry
¾ – 1 tsp ground cumin – I like things spicy, so all of these are higher than the original, but with a range for ya!
¾ – 1 tsp chili powder
½ tsp dry mustard
½ -3/4 tsp cinnamon
pinch of ground cloves
1 – 1 ½ Tbsp brown sugar
½ cup raisins
½ cup coarsely chopped stuffed green olives (In all my coarseness, I simply chop in half)
½ cup toasted slivered almonds (I use whole almonds from Costco and also cut in half – WAY cheaper than slivered almonds. I also do not toast out of laziness but it would probably make it even better to do this step)

If using turkey, brown in olive oil. If using lentils, cook them – allowing about 20 minutes for this – a great time to chop! Add onion, garlic and pepper to turkey(or, if using lentils, start fresh with olive oil) and sauté 3 – 5 minutes.

Add lentil to the sauée pot, or the sauté pot contents into the lentils. Add remaining ingredients and bring to a slow boil. Simmer for 15 – 20 minutes, uncovered. The lentils

Baby Steps to Better Health / Recipes: Entrees 186.

can thicken things up a bit, so if you need to, add a little more broth or water or more diced tomatoes with juice to reach the desired thickness. I serve this with either rice or cornbread. You don't have to serve it with anything because it totally rocks, to quote my 11 year old.

POWER TABBOULEH (GF/V)
- adapted from Deborah Madison's Bulgur and Green Lentil Salad with Chickpeas in *Vegetarian Cooking for Everyone*.

2 c chopped fresh parsley
2 c cooked quinoa (or whatever grain you have on hand)
1 ½ c cooked French lentils (I'm sure brown would be fine too, but I do like the green here)
1 bay leaf (opt.)
1 c cooked or canned garbanzo beans (drain and rinse if canned)
zest of two lemons
2 cloves garlic, made very small however you like
4 scallions or spring onions, chopped small, including some green
½ c olive oil
6-8 Tbsp fresh lemon juice
1 tsp paprika
salt and pepper to taste

Cook lentils in boiling water with a bit of salt and a bay leaf. (I can't recommend this bay leaf maneuver enough – made the beans so flavorful and delish.) While the lentils cook, chop and combine all of the cold solid ingredients. Drain the lentils and let them cool for about half an hour (unless you want your tabbouleh warm). Add the lentils to the chopped ingredients. Combine lemon juice, oil and paprika and pour it on. Toss everything to mix. Salt and pepper to taste. Can be served over or with a green salad

QUICK QUINOA STIR FRY (GF/V)
feel free to substitute and delete and re-do!! Spice amounts are approximate because I was dumping, not measuring… buyer beware.

Olive oil for pan
1 med-lge onion
1-2 cloves garlic
2 tsp. cumin seeds
2 tsp. ground cinnamon
3 med. Zucchini
3-4 med. Carrots
3-4 swiss chard leaves
1 cup raw cashews

2 cup dry quinoa
broth, stock, or water (for boiling quinoa)

Heat 4 cups water or stock. Heat oil in large skillet and add onions, crushed garlic, cumin seeds and cinnamon. When onion is transparent and cumin seeds are popping, add chopped carrots and zucchini. When water is boiling, add quinoa, stir, cover and turn heat down to low. Stir veggies occasionally and add swiss chard and cashews when carrots are softening. Salt as desired. Quinoa is done when water is absorbed and halos around individual grains are separating. Mix together or serve side by side with raisins on top if desired.

QUINOA POLENTA W/ TEMPEH SAUSAGE AND MUSHROOMS (GF/V)
- adapted from Isa Chandra Moskowitz's Millet Polenta and Tempeh Sausage recipes[81]

For the Polenta:

1 c quinoa
3 c vegetable stock or water (I used 1 stock, 2 water)
1 Tbsp olive oil plus more for pan
2 c fresh shredded greens (I used chard from my garden)
1 Tbsp fresh oregano (I grow it, but you could use 1/2 t dried)
½ tsp salt
dash of black pepper

For the Tempeh Sausage:

8 oz package tempeh
½ Tbsp fennel seed (yes, you need this if you want it to taste like sausage)
1 tsp dried basil
1 tsp dried marjoram or oregano
½ tsp red pepper flakes (opt – I left out for Ms. Picky Pants)
½ tsp dried sage
2 garlic cloves, crushed
2 Tbsp Bragg's or soy sauce
1 Tbsp olive oil
juice of ½ lemon

Sautéed Mushrooms:

mushrooms (I used about ½ lb)
olive oil for pan
dash salt

Start with the polenta as it needs some time to "set." Because of this requirement, this is also a great dish to make ahead of time. Toast the quinoa in a dry skillet for about 5 minutes until it browns a bit and becomes aromatic. Rinse several times in a sieve.

Bring water/broth, quinoa and olive oil to a boil in a pot. Lower heat and simmer for about 20 minutes (check on this to be sure it doesn't burn). Mix in greens, spices and continue to simmer on LOW for a few more minutes until liquid is absorbed. Scoop into an oiled dish – you can get fancy with this and make shapes, or you can do what I did and put it into a glass baking dish and cut it into shapes once firm. Allow to cool on counter.

Once the polenta is firm and cut, you will be browning your polenta shapes in a frying pan.
Give the polenta at LEAST an hour to cool if you are using a flat container, if you want to get real fancy shmancy and make a roll of polenta using a can as a mold, you'll need to let it cool for longer. When it is cool, cut it into whatever shapes you prefer. The rest of the elements of this dish will take about a half an hour.

Slice your mushrooms, warm olive oil in the pan, spread mushroom slices (or chunks if you prefer) in the pan. Sprinkle with salt. Leave them alone until the mushrooms are wet on top and starting to curl under, then flip them. While the mushrooms are sautéing, crumble the tempeh into a pan and add enough water to near cover it. Simmer the tempeh over med-high until most water is absorbed or for about 12-15 minutes. Assemble the herbs and seasoning for the sausage in a bowl. Drain remaining water from tempeh, return tempeh and seasonings to pan until a little brown (about 10 minutes). Don't forget about your mushrooms. When they are browned to your liking, remove them from the pan and set aside. Add a little olive oil, and put polenta into the frying pan. Brown for a few minutes on each side.

Serve by placing polenta on plate, sprinkling sausage on top of it, decorating with sautéed mushrooms, and sprinkling with any leftover bits of greens that didn't make it into the polenta. Add some toasted nuts if you're feeling a little EXTRA fancy.

RAW ZUCCHINI WOMANICOTTI (GF/V)

2 medium sized zucchini
1 c filling as described below
herbed olive oil as below
fresh tomatoes

To prepare the zucchini I used a mandoline. I suppose you could do it by hand, but that would require far greater knife skills than I possess and I am quite sure I would truly cut my finger off then. At any rate, you want the zucchini cut lengthwise in a thickness that you could conceivably roll. Lightly salt the zucchini and let it set a while so some of the

Baby Steps to Better Health / Recipes: Entrees   189.

water comes out – will help with the rolling. Blot zucchini dry. Plop an amount that looks sensible in the middle of the roll and wrap the sides around it. Drizzle with oil and tomatoes.

Cheeze Filling

1 c sunflower cheez (in our appetizers and dippers section – leave out the dill)
1 c moxerella[82] cheese (vegan mozzarella cheese – recipe link below)

Put in food processor. Blitz. Done.

Herbed Olive Oil

½ c olive oil
small handful basil

I put these into a blender and made lovely green herby oil, but there's no reason you couldn't chop the basil and add it to the oil by hand.

The family verdict on this raw zucchini dish? The adults watched in horror as the children had seconds, limiting our potential scarfing.

ROCKIN' GLUTEN FREE FALAFEL (GF/V)
– adapted from Isa Chandra Moskowitz' falafel found in *Vegan with a Vengeance*

1/3 c gluten free rolled oats
2 c cooked chickpeas (canned is fine, just drain and rinse)
2 Tbsp chickpea flour
1 medium onion, chopped
¾ tsp garlic powder (can sub 1 -2 cloves fresh)
½ tsp baking powder
½ tsp ground cumin (more for folks with cumin love)
1 tsp ground coriander
¼ tsp of cayenne (or 1/8 tsp white pepper)
¼ c chopped fresh parsley
½ tsp salt
vegetable oil for frying (I used olive oil, but will use safflower next time)
large leaf lettuce
falafel fixings (chopped tomato, cukes, whatever floats your boat)
tahini dressing

Put the oats in a food processor and pulse until the oats look more like bread crumbs than oats. Add chickpeas and pulse until chickpeas are chopped. Add all ingredients through the salt and process until you have a cohesive, but somewhat coarse mixture. It will be a little green from the parsley – it's okay. You may want to stop the machine and scrape down the sides of the bowl a couple of times. Remove bowl of food processor (with blade inside) and put in the fridge (with the cover on) for at least ½ an hour.

When the time is right, form the batter into 2 inch patties about ½ inch thick. Warm oil in the bottom of a pan (I used my cast iron and it worked supah). Use more oil than a low fat cook would normally use, but probably avoid the ½ inch recommended in the original because I thought that was gross. I know falafel are traditionally deep fried -- my shallow fried falafel were fab. When oil is warm (shimmery and bubbles up a little when a little batter is added), place patties in pan. Flip after a couple of minutes, watching for browning. Remove to drain on paper towels or paper bag you wish to reuse. Serve with fixins.

SAVORY VEGAN (or not) PANCAKES (V Option)

These are great when you have an odd assortment of items that you'd like to tie together in about a half an hour. Our savory pancakes were topped with roasted asparagus, chickpeas, grape tomatoes, corn, leftover vegan cheese sauce, and some spring onions.

1.5c whole wheat flour
.5c corn meal
2tsp baking powder
1tsp baking soda
1.5tsp salt
1tsp herbs – whatever matches your toppings best (optional, I skipped because they don't like "green things" in their food and will destroy a pancake picking a fleck out)
2c non-dairy milk (or moo juice if you drink it)
2 flax eggs (or chicken, if you eat them)
4Tbsp olive oil (part of what makes them savory, you see)

Procedure is the same as for other pancakes. Warm skillet in oven at 325. Make flax egg and chill. Mix dry, mix wet (add chilled flax egg). Combine wet and dry. Let rest 10 minutes. Scoop with 1/4c measure into pre-warmed skillet on medium stove. WATCH for firm edges and a few bubbles. Flip. Keep warm in oven. I served all toppings separate as this works better for my small people, but it does make a pretty plate to assemble the items before serving.

So now you know, the possibilities are endless. Mexican pancakes, Italian pancakes… whatever your leftovers and random bits suggest to you. Pancakes make it possible… at least they do in my house

SINGAPORE NOODLES w/ BAKED TOFU (GF/V)

For the baked tofu:
1 block extra firm tofu with excess water squeezed out
Marinade:
1.5 Tbsp roasted sesame oil
2 Tbsp Bragg's liquid aminos or soy sauce
juice from 1 lime
1/8 tsp. chili powder (I used chipotle which is strong – you might like more if using standard chili powder)

Save any leftover marinade to add to the whole dish at the end.

To bake the tofu:

Put parchment paper on a baking sheet. Slice your tofu about 1/4" thick and lay the slices on the tray. Brush the marinade on the top of the slices and bake at 375 for 10 minutes. Flip the slices and re-apply marinade. Put back in oven for 5 – 10 minutes and flip again if you like. Keep in oven until you reach desired toughness / chewiness. Cut some of the slices into cubes to put over noodles (recipe below). The whole slices make a nice sandwich.

Noodles:

1 pack thin rice stick noodles (rice vermicelli)
1 red or green bell pepper (or half of each) – thinly sliced
1 carrot into match stick size bits
3 c Napa cabbage (shredded)
3 tsp minced ginger
2 green onions or one small leek

Then for the sauce mix together:

1/8 – 1/4 cup water or broth
1 teaspoon brown sugar (or favorite sweetener)
1/2 tsp salt (or 1 tsp soy sauce)
1 1/2 Tbsp curry powder, or to taste

Prepare noodles according to package directions, drain and set aside. Then in a skillet or a wok, heat some oil then add, scallions, sugar, ginger – then peppers, carrots and lastly cabbage. Add a little water to help cook down the cabbage. Drain the noodles and chop. Mix with veggies and then add the remainder of the tofu marinade and taste. I added another Tbsp or so of Bragg's (or soy sauce) at this point. Serve with some of the tofu pieces. As an option, top with pineapple or orange chunks.

SLOW & SIMPLE, TORTILLAS, BEANS AND RICE (V)
- adapted from Deborah Madison's *Vegetarian Cooking for Everyone*

Whole Wheat Tortillas

2 c whole wheat flour
1 tsp salt
1 ½ tsp baking powder
2 tsp olive oil
¾ c water

Mix flour, salt and baking powder in bowl. Sprinkle in oil and mix with your hands to combine.
Add water and mix with your hands to combine. Form into a ball. Let rest for 15 minutes. On floured surface, divide ball into 8 equal portions. Roll each portion into a ball.

One at a time, roll out each ball as thin as you can. Use a rolling pin. Roll top to bottom, side to side, on the diagonal one way and then the other. Or let your six year old do it and let go of the desire for circular tortillas. If stickiness causes problems, add a dusting of flour. Add flour between tortillas. While rolling the last few, turn the stove on under a pan – about medium heat.
Let the pan get good and hot.

Place the tortillas in the pan one at a time. Let the tortilla cook for about a minute and then flip.
Cook about a minute and remove from the heat. Next tortilla. Stack finished tortillas on a plate and keep in warm oven or keep under cover until you're ready to eat.

Easy Peasy Rice and Beans

cooked brown rice in adequate quantity (cook with veggie stock or broth for extra yum)
black beans (soaked and cooked or if canned, drained and rinsed)
chopped red onion in amount that will give oomph without overwhelming
shake of cumin
shake of chipotle
shake of salt
chopped cilantro
1 Tbsp fresh lime juice
drizzle olive oil

Combine. Stir. Done.

Serve with chopped fresh veggies and chimmichurri (in sauce section) or salsa.

SPINACH CHICKPEA BURGERS (GF/V)
- adapted from a recipe by James Thresher in *The Washington Post*[83]

5 ounces fresh spinach (other greens, like kale and chard work as well)
oil for the pan
1 ¾ c cooked chickpeas (drained and rinsed if you're using canned), divided
2 flax eggs (chickie eggs work too)
1 tsp salt
2 Tbsp lemon juice
½ - ¾ c chickpea flour (other flours work here as well, but the flavor of the chickpea is great, and it works for those trying to cut back on gluten)

Warm a pan on the stove with just a drizzle of your preferred oil. Add spinach and stir. Cook only until spinach (or whatever green you've chosen) is wilted. Don't go farther. Catch it while it's still bright green and beautiful. Remove to a sieve and allow wilted greens to drip in the sink to remove excess water.

Add 1 ½ c chickpeas, eggs, salt, and lemon juice to the food processor and blitz until your mixture is about the consistency of a chunky hummus. Remove to mixing bowl. Press on spinach with spoon to press out any remaining excess water. Add spinach and remaining ¼ c chickpeas to the batter and use a potato masher or large spoon to incorporate these ingredients.
Add chickpea flour until the batter can be molded with your hands into patties that are still a little wet, but will hold together. Add oil to pan to warm.

Create patties with batter. Our single batch made 3 adult sized and 3 kid sized burgers. It's really not that important that you get the sizing right – it is YOUR dinner, after all. Place patties in warm pan and allow to brown. Flip after 5-8 minutes and brown the other side. Once brown, lower heat to keep warm until you are ready to serve, or place in warm oven. They are very tolerant of being "overdone." Very nice with cumin tinted mayo (or vegan version)

SUMMER AWESOMNESS FRITTERS WITH TOMATO AND AVOCADO (V Option)
- makes enough for several adults for one meal or two adults for one dinner and a few lunches

5 c shredded zucchini, drained
1 c grits (I used semolina, but would use grits or coarse corn meal next time)
1 ½ c whole wheat flour
½ all purpose flour
¼ c nutritional yeast or parmesan
½ tsp Old Bay seasoning
4 tsp salt (or less if you're not like me)

1 tsp baking powder
4 eggs (I used flax)
2 c buttermilk (I used soured almond milk)
2 c corn (preferably leftover amazing grilled corn)
1 ½ c fresh chopped tomato
1 Tbsp chopped fresh basil
1 T chopped fresh parsley
½ avocado cut into pieces
drizzle rice vinegar
drizzle balsamic

Prep Notes: Shred your zucchini, either in a food processor or using a grater. Place in colander or sieve and salt lightly. Allow to sit (in the sink) for at least fifteen minutes. Your zucchini will drop a lot of water and your fritters will be lighter and better cooked through than if you skip this step, trust me. If you're making flax eggs, this is a good time to go ahead and get on that as well. Soured almond milk? Sounds gross, yes, and frankly, it wasn't pretty, but it did the job. I used a 2c measure, put 2 T of white vinegar in the bottom and then filled to 2c with UNSWEETENED PLAIN almond milk. Got all curdly and separated a bit, still worked just fine and tasted superb (I mean in the fritters, no I'm not that hardcore, I did NOT drink the soured almond milk).

In a large bowl, combine flours, yeast or cheese, Old Bay and salt. For those of you who aren't from around these parts: if you haven't heard of Old Bay, I am VERY, VERY sorry. It is a seasoning mix that is used in this area, mostly in seafood dishes, and in particular on steamed blue crabs. If you don't have any in your area (and again, this would be VERY sad), I imagine you could sub out some other spice blend intended for the steaming of seafood. You could also leave it out, but you'd be missing out on some awesome. Stir to combine. Press the top of the pile of zucchini to release more liquid. I've even gone so far as to wrap it in a tea towel at this point and squeeze more liquid out… this was probably unnecessary, but kind of cool to see.

Add eggs and buttermilk or soured milk to dry ingredients. Stir to combine without over mixing. Add zucchini and corn and gently stir to distribute. Let rest for 10 or 15 minutes. Cook as you would pancakes. For me this means a cast iron skillet on medium with vegetable oil heated in the bottom. Flip when firm on edges and some bubbles have formed. Cook in batches and keep warm in oven.

While cooking fritters, assemble avocado tomato goodness by combing the remaining ingredients. Serve fritter with tomato avocado goodness on top

SUNFLOWER LEMON PESTO on SPAGHETTI SQUASH (GF/V)

Pesto:

1 c soaked sunflower seeds (soak them in water overnight or for about 6 hours and rinse well)
1/8 – ¼ c water
juice from 1 to 2 lemons
1 medium to large clove garlic
¾ tsp salt
2 handfuls fresh basil
black pepper to taste

To ensure that garlic is mixed in evenly you may choose to press the garlic, or to chop it with the processor blade first, but in general you want to put everything but the basil in the food processor and wrangle it all together. Then add basil and mix it until as finely chopped as you desire. If your mixture is too thick add a little more water until you are satisfied with the texture.

Spaghetti Squash:

Cook a medium to large spaghetti squash by cutting it in half lengthwise and placing it boiling water for about 15- 20 minutes or until tender. The skin becomes a little more translucent when it is cooked through at which point you carefully, and using pads of some sort – it's hot – hold the squash and scrape out the lovely strands that resemble spaghetti. Place a pile of squash in a bowl with a schmop of sunflower pesto on top

SUSHI SALAD or SUSHI IN A BOWL (GF/DF)

what you need to make a sushi salad (if you like cold) or a sushi bowl (if you like it hot) is:

- sheets of nori (paper like seaweed)
- sticky, slightly sweet rice
- wasabi (which can be purchased as a powder or a paste)
- soy sauce or Bragg's liquid aminos
- some type of fish like product: I used lox. (I used to use fake crab meat but am uncomfortable with the product now – but it's your call!) You could also use cooked shrimp, or if you are really brave, raw tuna or something. I don't go there because I took parasitology back in my undergraduate days.
- fresh crispy vegetables like cucumbers, carrots, peppers,
- avocado is a delightful addition to this
- and if you like, some lightly sautéed greens.

Sticky, slightly sweet rice:
these measurements were for our family of 3 and I always make leftovers, so adjust to your needs.

1 ½ c dry rice, cooked according to package directions (there are sushi rices, I use brown, long grain)
1 ½ Tbsp rice vinegar
1 ½ Tbsp sugar

Cook the rice as normal and when it's getting close to done, heat the vinegar and sugar on low to melt and combine. After the rice has absorbed the water, add the mixture and stir.If you choose, sauté some greens in a touch of your fave oil with a smidge of sesame oil. I used kale and I also threw in some sesame seeds. Now either let the rice and greens cool or proceed for warm sushification.

Chop your veggies into salad sized chunks (avocado is HIGHLY recommended). Mix your wasabi powder to package directions. You can then add it some soy sauce or Bragg's to make a little dressing. This is a very personal mixing as wasabi is hot and different products will pack different punches. Try mixing a little of the two and then tasting with a little rice. Set aside.

Mix ingredients to your hearts content, making sure to sneak some of the greens into little people's bowls under the rice ;-). Add torn pieces of nori as you pile in ingredients. If you add it all at one time you will get chunks of nori which most people probably won't care for. After all is in the bowl carefully apply soy or Bragg's with or without wasabi.

SWEET POTATO CRUSTED QUICHE (GF/V)
inspired by Claire at Just Blither Blather[84]

Crust:

3 cups shredded sweet potato (I used the food processor)
A drizzle of olive oil

Preheat oven to 375.
Mix sweet potato and a little olive oil and press into a 9 – 10" pie plate
Bake for 15 minutes

Filling:

1 onion, chopped
1 clove of garlic, minced
oil for sauté
2 cups of vegetable of choice (I used shredded broccoli stem and some leeks)

salt and pepper to taste
6 eggs
Splash of water

Sauté the onions and garlic until translucent. Add the other veggies you are using and cook until a little tender. Add salt and pepper to taste (the original recipe uses collards which sounds lovely!). Place veggies in crust after crust comes out of the oven. Beat the eggs and splash of water together and pour over veggies. Bake at 375 for 35 – 45 minutes or until set.

SWEET POTATO PATTIES with BLACK BEANS AND GREENS (GF/V)

The Black Beans

olive oil for the pan
½ small onion, chopped fine
2 ½ c cooked black beans or 2 cans, drained and rinsed
½ c water
1 tsp Bragg's or soy sauce
1 tsp dried oregano
dash garlic powder

In a small pot, warm olive oil on low-medium heat. Add onions and cook for a few minutes, stirring periodically. When onions are translucent, add the other ingredients and simmer over low heat while you prepare the rest of the meal. Stir occasionally to prevent sticking. Add water if necessary to get the consistency you prefer.

The Patties

2 ½ c sweet potato (cooked until VERY soft)
1 c cooked grain (I used quinoa)
1 ½ c chickpea flour
1 tsp salt
1 c rolled oats
1 tsp orange zest
½ tsp paprika
¼ tsp garlic powder
olive oil for the pan

Mix all ingredients in a large bowl. Warm oil in the pan at slightly less than medium heat. Preheat the oven to 225. Use a mixing or soup spoon to spoon large dollops (sorry for the technical term) into the pan. Allow to cook for about 5 minutes per side, or until brown. Flip and brown the other side. Transfer to a baking dish and allow to rest in oven while cooking the rest of the patties.

The Greens

olive oil for the pan
about 8 ounces of your preferred dark green leafy
1 clove garlic, minced
toasted nuts (opt)

Warm the olive oil on low-medium. Add minced garlic and cook until fragrant (about 30 seconds). Add greens and cook until wilted, stirring to ensure all greens make contact with the hot part of the pan. Remove from heat when they are just starting to look ready. Add nuts (we used walnuts).

When it was all said and done, we served the beans over the patties, added a dollop of Annie's cashew cream[85], a spoon of our favorite salsa, and added the greens to the plate. The dish tasted best when all the elements were on the fork together, regardless of what Ms. Picky Pants (who would dearly love to have a plate with sections) says.

TOFU BAHN MI: VIETNAMESE PLANT STRONG (GF/V)
- inspired by Meatless Monday Site[86]

If you need to cook rice you will want to time starting that between pickling the carrots and starting the tofu sauté.

Quick Pickled Asian Carrots

2 c carrots julienned (or just sliced thin and pretty)
1 c rice wine vinegar
3 Tbsp coconut sugar (or your sweetener of choice)
1 tsp salt

To prepare the carrots, simply mix the pickling brine in a 2 c measuring cup (or wherever you want). Arrange the carrots in a non-reactive dish that is small enough to force the brine to cover the carrots. Pour brine over. Marinate anywhere from 1.5 hours to 3 days ;-).

Marinated Tofu

1 block firm or extra firm tofu, pressed for at least 30 minutes*
3 Tbsp soy sauce or Bragg's
2 Tbsp rice vinegar
½ tsp lemongrass (to taste and if you can get fresh, rock it out)
2 cloves of garlic minced
2 tsp coconut sugar or sweetener of choice

Tofu does NOT need a lot of time to marinate - I would suggest 15 minutes to half an hour TOPS. Slice your tofu into 8 rectangles – I went the short way – if you go long your cooking time may be shorter as the slices will be thinner. Place rectangles in non-reactive dish. Mix marinade ingredients in a small bowl, or container with a spout if you're like me and tend toward messes in the kitchen. Pour over tofu. Let marinate.

Heat your preferred high heat oil in a pan over med-high heat. Do more than grease the pan – be more generous with the oil than you might otherwise be inclined to do, but do NOT pour a deep fry amount. When the oil is warm, add tofu. Now for the hard part of cooking tofu, let it be.
If you try to check on it or flip it too soon, you will have a disintegrating stuck on mess. Let it be, let it brown a bit – then flip it. You'll have to time this according to the thickness of your cuts, but I would count on at least 5 minutes per side.
I let mine go longer and I really liked the results.

To Make it a Meal:

Cucumbers, green peppers, avocado (or raw veggies of your choice)
sesame seeds
cilantro
freshly cooked rice or warmed up leftover rice

Serve all together over rice!

VARIA-BOWL (GF/DF/V depending on what you choose)

As is our practice here on the pantry, I'm now going to throw a series of general recommendations at you that when I follow them, result in dinner. For a nutritious and delicious varia-bowl, prepare:
a grain or noodle,
a marinated or cooked green,
and chop several other veggies according to your preference.
I always add nuts for crunch and protein
and usually either parsley or cilantro for some yum.
Add seasonings to complement the cooked veggie. Easy, right?

I tend to serve these separately so everyone can construct their own version of the Varia-Bowl. They call this "deconstructed" in high cuisine circles; I call it sanity when dining with twin 5 year olds. Keeping all of the elements separate makes it much easier to accommodate the various preferences of my crew. They know they will still be having plenty of veggies, but they can skip one of them and the ones that they choose can sit on the plate without touching, as this seems to make them undesirable.

VEGGIE BURGER/ POTATO CAKE (GF/V)

1.5 cups of hummus (homemade is much cheaper!!)
1.5 cups of cooked lentils
3 cups cut, boiled potatoes (I used yukon gold that were on sale – but any potato will do)
½ cup brown rice flour
pinch of sage
½ Tbsp. ground cumin
1 medium onion, chopped
4 large handfuls baby spinach
touch of olive oil
½ tsp dried rosemary or 1 tsp fresh
salt and pepper to taste

Heat oven to 375. Line 2 cookie sheets with parchment paper. Mash 1st three ingredients into unity with a potato masher Ohm…. OHM… Whew – unity can be hard work ☺. Add brown rice flour, sage, cumin, salt and pepper. Heat olive oil in a pan, sauté rosemary and onion until onion is translucent, then add spinach just until it wilts and remove from heat. Add to dry ingredients.

Schmop large spoonfuls onto parchment paper lined baking trays and then tidy up a bit if you like tidy. Faster and neater than the make patties with the hands method. Place in oven and flip after 10 minutes. Cook for another 7 – 10 minutes or until desired doneness.

VEGGIES AU VIN (GF/V)
- adapted from Tofu Au Vin[87] on Meatless Mondays[88]

Olive oil for pans
1 ½ c onion, chopped
3 carrots, chopped
3 garlic cloves, minced or smashed
2 bay leaves
3 c red wine *
3 c water or veggie broth
2 Tbsp Braggs or soy sauce
1 Tbsp balsamic vinegar
1 c lentils (I used brown, but would use French next time)
18 oz mushrooms, rough cut
2 Tbsp corn starch
½ c water

salt and pepper to taste
1/3 c chopped parsley

Warm olive oil in large saucepan. Add onions and a sprinkle of salt and cook for about 5 minutes (stirring occasionally) on medium-low or until onions have become somewhat translucent. Add garlic and carrots and cook for another minute or two. Add bay leaves, wine and broth or water, soy and vinegar and bring to a boil. Add lentils, lower heat to simmer and cover. Cook for about 20 minutes or until lentils are tender.

While lentils cook, warm olive oil in a skillet. Add mushrooms and a sprinkle of salt. Sauté mushrooms until they are brown (let them sit still a bit to get good browning). A secret to browning mushrooms is not to put too many in the pan at once, "crowding the pan." Mushrooms release liquid as they cook; if you put them all in at once and they let all that water out, you'll end up boiling them instead of browning them – this is not a disaster, but I like mine browned. :-) As mushrooms brown, set them aside in a bowl. When lentils are tender, mix corn starch with water and add to lentil broth. Stir occasionally and cook for a few minutes until broth thickens. Add mushrooms to broth. Serve with your preferred grain. Add generous sprinkle of fresh parsley.

*The original recipe indicates that you could substitute broth with a little red wine vinegar for the wine in this recipe. I'm sure this would create a tasty dish, but am dubious about it evoking the same flavor profile. Bon Appétit!

WALDORF SAUTÉ (GF/V)

1 Tbsp coconut oil
1 sweet onion (med – large)
3 large ribs celery
2 – 3 cloves garlic (I used 2 large cloves)
2 tsp ground cumin
1 tsp salt
3 -4 c fresh spinach
1 large apple, cubed (I did not peel)
1 c walnuts
1 c peas (I used frozen)
2 – 3 red potatoes (optional)

Chop and mince your onion and garlic respectively (and respectfully). Chop celery. Heat coconut oil in a pan and sauté onion, garlic, celery and cumin until onion is a little translucent (nice to have it a bit crunchy with this dish). If using potatoes (I made once with and once without – nice either way) slice thinly and add at this point until tender. Add salt and spinach until the spinach is wilted. Add apple, walnuts and peas to warm. Serve over rice or other grain if desired – we enjoyed that vegetabl-y goodness all by itself!

WALNUT PESTO PASTA (GF/V)

1 lb. pasta of your choice (We used rice pasta to keep it GF)
3-4 cloves garlic
5-6 cups basil leaves – I filled my 9 cup Cuisinart about 3/4 full with basil leaves
2 c walnuts
1 – 2 Tbsp. oil- I used olive
1 tsp salt
1/4 cup nutritional yeast flakes. If you've never used them you're in for a treat, they bring a cheesy flavor to dairy free dishes (and also some selenium and zinc).
1 c & 2 Tbsp milk (I used homemade, unflavored almond)

Sauté the garlic in a spot of oil in a large pan which will later accommodate the rest of the sauce ingredients. Stuff the basil leaves, walnuts, salt, oil and 2 Tbsp. milk in Cuisinart and process, scraping down sides until consistency is smooth and there are no large chunks. Feel free to add a little more milk if you need it. Transfer mixture to sauté pan. Add the nutritional yeast flakes until all is incorporated and warm. Add more milk if needed. Mix half of this batch into a pound of pasta and freeze the rest for a quick and easy meal on another night. You could mix in vegetables, or serve them on the side. We served with broccoli and peas – some of us mixed in and some ate them on the side.

ZUCHEEZY NOODLES WITH CRUNCHY BITS (V Option)

1 lb noodles (I used whole wheat)
1 zucchini
½ c water
2 c soft cheese (Dairy or non-dairy)
milk to blend (Dairy or unsweetened non-dairy)
2 Tbsp nutritional yeast (opt.)
1 tsp salt
½ tsp garlic powder
1 ½ c unsweetened flake cereal/crackers/bread crumbs (opt)
½ c wheat germ (opt)
1 tsp kelp flakes (opt)

Preheat oven to 375. Lightly grease a casserole dish. For this little experiment, my kids chose gobetti (corkscrews) for this recipe (a little pretend democracy never hurts when trying a new recipe on them), but any thick noodle would work. Cook noodles according to package directions or your own tried and true.

While waiting for water to boil/noodles to cook, assemble your sauce. Peel zucchini and put in powerful blender (in whatever size your blender is going to need) and add enough water to create a slurry. Blend until the zucchini is unrecognizable. Add chunks of the soft cheese, adding milk to create motion in the blender and a very thick, but still pourable sauce consistency. Add nutritional yeast if you like it, and salt if you're not trying to avoid it. Add the garlic powder because it makes everything more awesome. Adjust spice and consistency to your tastes.

When noodles are done, drain them. Pour half into greased dish. Add half of your cheese sauce. Pour the rest of the noodles in and cover with the remaining sauce. Do not scrape out the blender – you will use the cheese on the sides for the topping.

The Topping: Measure the cereal and wheat germ into a bowl. Use a spoon to mash the cereal up a bit for easier eating. Add the scrapings from your sauce to give a little fat and damp to the crumb topping so it doesn't burn and actually gets a little crunch going. Add to top of casserole.

Bake in oven with rack in middle or just below (burned crumb topping is a buzzkill) for about a half an hour, or until it's hot enough for you, or until the children come completely unglued.

We served ours with peas (peas are always served with cheesy noodles here) and fresh carrots. Little buggers had no idea they were also eating zucchini until I revealed that at lunch today. They were unphased; I've no idea if that means they'll be open to zucchini, but I'm pretty sure I'll keep it a secret again next time and slip that bugger in there.

Salad Dressing

BASIC TAHINI SALAD DRESSING (V)
1 cup olive oil
1/4 cup tahini
1 1/2 Tbsp soy sauce or Bragg's liquid aminos
1 tsp honey
0-2 Tbsp water (taste it first and see if it's too strong and then temper with a little water)

Put all in a jar that is at least 14oz, with a good lid and shake it up.

FAT FREE SALAD DRESSING (V)

Rice Vinegar
Soy Sauce

That's it. Splash a little right on your salad. Mix 'em in a jar and taste then add more of the other one. Whatever. It's that simple.

HOMEY HONEY MUSTARD DRESSING (GF/V Option)

½ c plain yogurt (dairy or non) of your favorite type
1 Tbsp & 2 tsp maple syrup
1 Tbsp & 2 tsp dijon mustard (or try a different mustard!)
1 tsp apple cider vinegar (optional but a nice tang – stronger flavor)
pinch of salt

Mix all ingredients together. Pour it on your salad ;-)

MISO DRESSING (GF/V)

1 Tbsp yellow miso (would likely work with other kinds, but I can speak with authority on the yellow)
1 Tbsp Bragg's or soy sauce
2 Tbsp rice vinegar
1 Tbsp sesame oil

Combine ingredients and whisk until smooth. This dressing is light in flavor and works well with warm salads and more traditional fresh green salads.

Sauces

BASIL AVOCADO CREAM (V)
– inspired by this avocado pasta sauce dish[89].

1 ripe avocado
2 cloves garlic
handful fresh basil leaves
pinch of salt
juice of one lemon
twist of the pepper grinder

You know what's coming, right? Put it all in a food processor or blender. Process until smooth and creamy. Mix with pasta – this recipe would likely adequately cream up pasta for a few people. A little goes a long way. Top with pine nuts, or chopped nuts that you love. So incredibly awesome, and just the thing while you're watching your children scarf down their dinner, which does not include the suspicious green cream sauce. That's okay. I didn't want to share that night anyway. De-lish.

EASIEST TOMATO SAUCE EVER (V)
-adapted from Gena at Choosing Raw.com[90]

2 - 4 very large red or yellow bell peppers, deseeded
28 oz can of fire-roasted organic diced tomatoes
¼ cup sundried tomatoes
1 Tbsp olive oil
¼ tsp salt
Generous sprinkle dried thyme
Generous sprinkle dried oregano
Generous sprinkle of basil

Whiz this all together in your Vita-Mix or other strong blender til smooth and serve cold or warmed. I offered the masses their choice of thin, raw zucchini slices, whole wheat spaghetti or quinoa as the underlay for the sauce. It was very tasty and so fast it makes me tear up just thinking about it ;-).

FABU ASIAN PEANUT SAUCE (V)

Two large glops of peanut butter
A few shakes of soy or Bragg's (to taste)
red chili flakes (or chili paste)
crushed garlic
minced/crushed/or powdered ginger

chopped cilantro
water

This is a wonderful sauce in that it is highly adaptable and easy to adjust for different tastes and uses. I usually don't measure (shocker, I know), start with the PB, and add the other ingredients to taste (which means I get to eat it while I'm making it, which is obviously a good thing). Most of the ingredients are optional or could be changed out, but I find this combo to be the most yum. When I've mixed everything but the water to taste, I add enough water to make it suit my needs. If it's a drizzling sauce I add more water. If I want to dip veggies in it, less water. It keeps beautifully and adds a lovely Asian peanut vibe to just about anything you might want to eat. Great on noodles, fabulous on broccoli…. especially broccoli you've just brought in from the garden.

HARISSA (GF/V) North African sauce for roasted veggies, meat or whatever you like!!
- adapted from Saad Fayed[91]

2 Tbsp. garlic chili paste or sauce – I used a Vietnamese version
½ tsp salt
1 Tbsp olive oil
1 tsp ground coriander
1 tsp ground caraway seeds
½ tsp cumin

Grind and combine the spices in a coffee or spice grinder. (You can use already ground if you prefer, but my store did not offer ground caraway seeds.) Add chili garlic sauce and olive oil.

Use the sauce over roasted vegetables with couscous or quinoa or rice or to spice up any boring what's left in the fridge kind of meal!

HERBED BERRY SAUCE (GF/V)
- inspired by Emmy's Summer Berry Sauce[92]

¼ c water
1 tsp corn starch
2 Tbsp sugar
2 c berries (I used blackberries and blueberries)
juice of ½ lemon
6 small sprigs fresh thyme

Whisk water and corn starch together in small saucepan. Add sugar and berries and cook over medium heat. Stir occasionally to prevent sugar burning and to help berries

Baby Steps to Better Health / Recipes: Sauces   207.

break down. Add thyme and lemon juice, stir and allow syrup to simmer until it reaches a thickness you like. Sweet and tart and fabulously complex because of a few twigs thrown into the mix. Try on pancakes, ice cream, cake, yogurt, your finger....

KINDER, GENTLER CHIMICHURRI (GF/V)
– borrowed and slightly modified from Saveur's chimichurri

1 c parsley leaves
¾ c fresh cilantro leaves
¼ c fresh oregano leaves
¼ c red wine vinegar
6 cloves garlic
¼ poblano pepper
1 ½ tsp salt and ½ tsp pepper (or to taste)
½ c olive oil

Put everything but the olive oil into a food processor or blender. Drizzle the olive oil in while the machine is on. Put it on sandwiches, on roasted potatoes, on leftovers that were kind of bland, on a cauliflower steak (in vegan section).

LEMONY HUMMUS SAUCE or Combo Bowl Sauce (see Varia-Bowl) (GF/V)

1 cup of hummus (I used Lemony Roasted Garlic Hummus – in Appetizers and Dips section)
5 Tbsp nutritional yeast flakes
Juice of 2 lemons (about 6 Tbsp)
½ tsp garlic powder
½ tsp salt
¼ – ½ c water

Mix together.

NOT SO SOUR CREAM (V)
- adapted from everydaydishtv

1 ¾ c hemp seeds, cashews or pine nuts (I mixed them)
1 tsp apple cider vinegar
1 Tbsp soy sauce
¼ t salt
juice from a lemon
water as needed for consistency

Food processor. Fill it and leave on while you're doing anything else you can think of in the kitchen. When it's ready – creamy gooey smoothness. Use where you'd use sour cream….. or in creamy kale (in side dishes), vegan creamy biscuits (side dishes), or mix with salsa for a zippy dip, or a dippy zip!

PUMPKIN APPLE FIG BUTTER (GF/V)

1 cup of dried figs soaked overnight in 1 cup of water. (I'm thinking this would also be good with prunes, or other dried fruit)
6 cups chopped apples – I leave peels on – it's better for you and much less work.
1 and a half 15oz. can's pumpkin (about 3 cups puree if you're lucky enough to have the real thing)
1 Tbsp cinnamon
1 tsp allspice
¼ – ½ tsp ginger

Dump figs, soaking water and apples in the crockpot and cook on high for 4 hours. Stir about once an hour to prevent sticking and help the process along. Mash it up a bit and if it's not real soft, let it cook a bit longer. Puree. (I used a Vita Mix) Be careful – hot things can bubble , splatter and push the lid up and off!! Put back in the crockpot and add pumpkin and spices (or leave if you've used an immersion blender). Stir well and cook with lid off to desired consistency, stirring now and again. Thickening time will of course vary by taste and by how wet your pumpkin is.

PRUNE CARDAMOM SAUCE (GF/V)

This is an adaptation of <u>Date Cream</u> also found in this section. This is so easy that I'm embarrassed, but I can live with embarrassment I guess.

1/3 c prunes
2/3 c milk of choice (I used almond – don't think dairy would affect this negatively)
¼ tsp ground cardamom

Bring these 3 things into harmonious existence as a new and wonderful thing with a high speed blender. Perhaps a large food processor would work as well, but it is a bit wet. Adjust thickness to intent and taste. I think just a bit thicker than the above would be a good pairing with almond butter on a sandwich.

ROASTED ONION & FIG RELISH (GF/V)

1 lge sweet onion
1 lge red onion
8 fresh brown figs
1 Tbsp olive oil
2- 3 Tbsp balsamic
1/2 tsp salt

Pre-heat oven to 400. Lightly oil baking sheet with edges (I used the bottom of a broiler pan). Chop the onions fine – I used a food processor which left some big chunks using the top wheel, but I didn't want mush either. Might be better to chop fine by hand if you don't like a few big chunks. Add the figs to the food processor – or chop by hand into small bits. Mix together in a bowl and add oil, vinegar and salt. Spread out on baking sheet – it's pretty wet. Roast for about 30 minutes, stirring every 10 or so. It dries out a bit as it roasts so go until it is of a consistency you like. Your house will smell really great while this is going on! Put it on crackers, Mix a little into rice w/ some cheese. Use on a sandwich.

SIMPLE TOMATO SAUCE (GF/V)
- adapted from Deborah Madison *Vegetarian Cooking for Everyone*

2 Tbsp olive oil
1/4c chopped onion
2 cloves garlic, small (however you like to do it)
1 28 ounce can (or box) diced tomatoes (drained if you like really thick sauce)
1 tsp dry oregano
1 Tbsp fresh or 2 tsp dry basil
salt and pepper to taste

In a large skillet or pot, warm the oil over medium heat and sauté onion for about 5 minutes. Add garlic and cook until fragrant (about 30 seconds). Add tomatoes and simmer for 15 minutes or until the sauce is a thickness that suits you. Stir in oregano and basil (if dry) and simmer for and additional 5 minutes or so. If using fresh basil, add just before serving. Salt and pepper to taste. Run through blender or food processor if you like smooth sauce. We like it chunky. Serve over your favorite pasta, rice, quinoa, bulghur, any other grain you can think of. It's easy; it's awesome and it does NOT have anywhere near as much sugar as a Twinkie (as do some prepared tomato sauces). Bang, done.

WELCOME HOME VEGAN PESTO (GF/V)

Double batch sunflower cheez spread (omit the dill)
1 large clove garlic
6 cups packed fresh basil
1 t salt
6 Tbs olive oil

Follow the recipe for the sunflower cheez spread (to which I am now hopelessly and willfully addicted, by the way), omitting the dill (unless of course you like dill in your pesto), and adding a large clove of garlic. Process the cheez until it is as smooth as your patience will allow. Add the basil, additional salt and the olive oil and process again until ingredients are incorporated.

The pesto will not be as green as traditional pesto, but like traditional pesto, it WILL oxidize, so the color will go from green to brown when left uncovered or as time passes. Stir for better color. This recipe makes A LOT of pesto. Freeze some for an easy meal later!

Sides

AWESOME OVEN FRIES (GF/V)
Adapted from the Weight Watchers New Complete Cookbook
1.25 lbs potatoes, peeled (if you must) and cut to 1/2" fry shapes
¾ to 1tsp salt
½ tsp sugar
4 tsp oil
1 tsp paprika
¼ tsp pepper (I use white to avoid kid detection)

Preheat oven to 450. Lightly grease baking sheets or line with parchment paper (works better). Combine potatoes, 1/4t salt, sugar and cold water to cover. Soak 15 minutes, drain &blot dry. In dry bowl, combine potatoes with oil, paprika and pepper. Arrange in single layer on baking sheet. Bake, turning as they brown. 35-45 minutes. Sprinkle with salt. Voila. Fan-flipping tastic. Yes, you should probably make a double batch.

CHEMICAL FREE SIMPLY FABU SWEET AND SOUR PICKLES (GF/V)

1 large English style or 2 medium whatever you have on hand cucumbers
1/4 onion cut into slices (or however your crew will eat them)
2 c water
4Tbsp sugar
1/2 c apple cider vinegar
1/2tsp celery seeds
3tsp salt
1tsp mustard seeds

Slice cucumber however you like. Put cukes and onions in bowl that will hold your cukes and some liquid – ideally to cover cukes. Bring water just to a boil and add sugar – take off heat to avoid scalding sugar and stir to dissolve sugar. Add other ingredients and stir. Allow to cool for a few minutes. Pour over cukes and allow to sit for at least half an hour. Longer would be better and a chill would be nice too. We ate ours at room temp and straight out of the bowl until all that was left was the brine. De-lish and no high fructose corn syrup or Yellow 5 in sight.

COOL SUMMER VEGGIE QUINOA (GF/V)

3 cups cooked quinoa (or whatever amount will work for you)
2 cucumbers, rough cut
2 c rough cut tomatoes
2 Tbsp olive oil
4 tsp white wine vinegar
salt and pepper to taste

1 tsp oregano
fresh chopped parsley (opt)

Quinoa must be rinsed before cooking to taste at all palatable. The quinoa seeds are coated in saponins, vegetable substances, that make quinoa taste bitter. I soak mine in a bowl or pot and then drain through a fine strainer. After rinsing, add quinoa to boiling water (2 cups water for every one cup quinoa) and allow to simmer for about 15 minutes or until liquid is absorbed. When quinoa is done cooking, chill in the refrigerator so as not to cook those tremendous raw veggies in the bowl. When mealtime is 5 minutes away, add cut veggies to chilled quinoa. Sprinkle in olive oil (more if you like) and white wine vinegar. Season with salt, pepper, and oregano. Stir.

CREAMED KALE (GF/V)

olive oil for pan
large clove garlic, mashed or minced
giant bunch of kale, de-stemmed and ripped into smaller pieces
1/4 c Not So Sour Cream

Warm oil in pan. Sauté garlic until you can breathe it. Turn heat down a little (below medium is good). Add kale, sprinkle with a bit of salt and cover with lid to improve the wilting for the top leaves. Stir occasionally to prevent overcooking. When wilt is done, lower heat further and add NSSC and stir to distribute and warm through.

DIJON ROASTED GARLIC BRUSSELS SPROUTS (GF/V)

Brussels Sprouts – enough to about cover the bottom of your baking pan
½ – 1 Tbsp oil
salt to taste
1 ½ - 2 ½ tsp dijon mustard
1 tsp balsamic vinegar
4 cloves roasted garlic
1 tsp oil

Wash the Brussels sprouts, cut the tough stem end off and then cut the brussels in half. Toss with the ½ – 1 Tbsp oil (I used avocado – your favorite or what you have on hand will work as well) and salt. Spread out on a baking pan, and roast at 375. They usually take about 30 – 40 minutes.
While they are roasting mash the garlic, vinegar, tsp of oil and mustard together. When the Brussels have just about reached their desired tenderness, take them out and mix in the sauce. Roast for another 5 – 10 minutes.

GARLIC MUSHROOMS (GF/V)
– inspired by Perfect Vegetarian[93]

5 T olive oil
4 cloves garlic, chopped fine
1 lb of mushrooms, I used cremini
salt, to taste
3 Tbsp chopped parsley
1 Tbsp fresh lemon juice
pepper, to taste

To prepare mushrooms, clean them as you prefer. Trim the stems to the length you prefer. I don't find anything wrong with a little stem on a cooked mushroom, so I don't take the whole thing. For this dish larger mushrooms should be cut in half or even quarters. Warm the olive oil in the pan over medium heat. Add the garlic and cook until fragrant (about 30 seconds). Add mushrooms and sauté with a little stirring until the mushrooms have soaked up all the olive oil (yes, they'll take it all). Turn heat to low, add some salt to the mushrooms and continue to cook for another 5-10 minutes or until the mushrooms have released their liquid. Raise heat to medium-high. Add parsley, lemon juice, and salt and pepper to taste. Cook for another minute or so, stirring a lot. Remove from heat.

SIMPLE, NOT PLAIN, GREEN BEANS (GF/V)

enough green beans for your tribe with an extra handful or two for leftover lunches, with ends trimmed
olive oil for the pan (about 1 Tbsp, you're not frying them)
sprinkle of salt
toasted pecans (or nuts of preference, you can also do raw, but the toasted are super special)

Toast nuts while trimming the beans by warming a cast iron pan (with no oil in it). When the pan is warm, put the pecans in and let them sit for a minute. While trimming the beans, stir the pecans around occasionally, and attempt to flip them over so they are toasted on both sides
If you smell the nuts while you're trimming your beans, you should stir them. The scent gets stronger and more wonderful just before they burn. On to the beans!

Warm olive oil in pan. Add green beans and let them be for a couple of minutes. As the beans release some moisture you'll hear noises that sound like frying, but it's not. Treat them like the nuts – flip them around occasionally, keep your eye on them. They will get brighter green.
Sprinkle a little salt and remove to serving dish when they are warm, but still entirely and delightfully solid. Add pecans, toss, eat.

GREENS BEANS – FANCY SHMANCY (GF/V)

Fancy Shmancy Green Beans or Green Beans with Pecans, Clementines and Balsamic Vinegar

enough beans for your tribe
olive oil for the pan
sprinkle of salt
toasted pecans
2 chopped clementines (or other sweet orange)
1 small glug balsamic vinegar

Toast nuts as in previous recipe. Peel and segment clementines. Toast nuts while trimming the beans by warming a cast iron pan (with no oil in it). When the pan is warm, put the pecans in and let them sit for a minute. While trimming the beans, stir the pecans around occasionally, and attempt to flip them over so they are toasted on both sides. If you smell the nuts while you're trimming your beans, you should stir them. The scent gets stronger and more wonderful just before they burn. On to the beans!

Warm olive oil in pan. Add green beans and let them be for a couple of minutes. As the beans release some moisture you'll hear noises that sound like frying, but it's not. Treat them like the nuts – flip them around occasionally, keep your eye on them. They will get brighter green.
Sprinkle a little salt and remove to serving dish when they are warm, but still entirely and delightfully solid. Add nuts, clementines, and a small glug of balsamic vinegar.

GRILLED CORN AND FRESH TOMATO SUMMER CRUDO (GF/V)

Kernels cut from 3 ears of grilled corn*
2 large or three medium tomatoes, chopped coarsely
1 can (drained, rinsed) or 1.5 cups cooked chickpeas
3 handfuls fresh spinach chopped coarsely
1 small handful fresh basil chopped
a couple of handfuls of leftover peas (or whatever you have lurking in your fridge)
juice of 1 lemon
1 tsp salt
1 Tbsp olive oil
fresh ground pepper to taste
1-2 cloves garlic, made small however you like

No great complication here. Just put it all in a bowl and stir gently to combine without destroying the tomatoes. Top with sunflower cheese or parmesan if you like.

HERBED SWEET TOMATOES WITH RICE (GF/V)

2 cups brown rice (cooked in vegetable broth for extra flavor)
1 Tbsp olive oil
1 medium onion (sweet if you have it!)
1-2 cloves garlic (I used 1 large clove)
2 med or 1 lge zucchini cut how you like (I slice coins and then cut coins into strips)
3-4 cups sweet little 'maters
Optional – other fresh veggies – SWEET peppers are especially good
1 Tbsp fresh oregano (1 tsp dried)
½ c chopped fresh parsley
¼ – ½ c chopped fresh basil (I hold a stack of leaves and cut strips with scissors)
chopped walnuts
salt and pepper to taste

Set the water (or broth) boiling for rice. Chop onion and mince or crush garlic. Cook onion and garlic in large skillet in oil until transparent, or even browning a bit. Chop zucchini and tomatoes (I just cut my little maters in half). Add zucchini and oregano and cook until desired tenderness

Add tomatoes just to warm them up. Remove from heat and stir in parsley and basil. Serve over rice. Top with chopped walnuts as desired – I used about 2 Tbsp in my bowl because they are SO good. Add more basil and parsley if it doesn't have enough Ka-Pow.

MASHED & ROASTED, or ABUSED CAULIFLOWER (GF/V)

6 medium red potatoes cut into chunks (I always leave skins on)
1 smallish head of cauliflower, also cut into chunks (see the abuse begins already)
4 plump garlic cloves, peeled and cut in half
1 sprig (about 4") of fresh rosemary clipped into little pieces (about ½ Tbsp – or 1 tsp dried)
2 – 4 Tbsp olive oil. Use more than you might for plain roasting so the mix will be nice and greasy for mashing.
salt and pepper to taste
½ – 1 cup unsweetened milk of your favorite variety. I used homemade almond milk.

Preheat oven to 400. Place all but milk in a bowl or right on a baking tray and mix it up. Roast for about 30 minutes or until very tender (times will vary by chunk size and crowding). Place in high powered blender (I use a Vita Mix) and pour in milk a bit at a time until as creamy as desired. You may have to complete the mashing in a bowl if it is too thick for your blender. Next time I think I'll use my hand held beaters, or just be more liberal with the milk from the get go to avoid overheating my Vita Mix.

MEDITERRANEAN WILTED GREENS (GF/V)

4 c geens, roughly chopped (I used kale)
2 tsp balsamic vinegar
2 tsp olive oil
1 small clove garlic
1 Tbsp pine nuts (or really whatever nut you have that you like)
2 tsp raisins or currants (optional)

I'm betting you can guess what to do here. Throw everything but the pine nuts and raisins if you use them in a bowl and massage or toss. The thicker your greens, the more you should mix, and the more time you want to give it to marinate (20-30 mins). When done, add pine nuts and raisins (if you choose). I served mine with whole wheat shells and garbanzo beans. Delish.

How else could we change it? A French version of the Mediterranean greens might use wine vinegar and add a bit of fresh thyme and parsley. A Japanese version of the original namul might use rice vinegar instead of soy sauce, and come with a side of wasabi, or have nori flakes broken into it.

MOO-LESS, FLAVOR-FULL PARMESAN SPRINKLES (GF/V)
-adapted from Angela Liddon's vegan parmesan cheez[94]

½ c raw sunflower seeds
¾ c raw sesame seeds
¼ c nutritional yeast flakes
½ tsp salt

Place all ingredients in blender. Blend until powdery – don't go too long or the sunflower seeds will start to turn into sunflower butter!Place on top of pasta... or other things as well!

MUNG BEAN SPROUT NAMUL (GF/V)
adapted from Ani Phyo's recipe in *Ani's Raw Food Asia*

4 c mung bean sprouts
2 Tbsp apple cider vinegar
2 Tbsp sesame oil
1 tsp maple syrup
1 small clove garlic, made small however you like
1 tsp salt
1 tsp minced ginger
large pinch red pepper or chili flakes

Doesn't get much easier than this kind of procedure. Put all in bowl, toss. Wait 20 minutes or so. Eat. Love. We had ours as a side to veggie burgers at lunch, but I could easily see adding it to the top of any Asian dish with crunchy scrumptious results. While I must confess the kids wouldn't touch this one, I should also say that I was glad, deep inside, that I got to eat that much more.

NATURALLY SWEET SWEET POTATOES (GF/V)
– inspired by Roasted Sweet Potatoes and Bananas[95] at the Mayo Clinic website

1 pound sweet potatoes, scrubbed, ends and any odd bits trimmed, chopped into 1 inch pieces
1 ½ tsp olive oil
¼ tsp salt
juice of 1 orange
1/8 tsp cinnamon
pinch cayenne
2 bananas, peeled and cut into 1 inch rounds

Preheat oven to 450. Toss cut potatoes in olive oil and salt. Place on baking tray (I lined mine with parchment because I am lazy) and roast in oven on middle rack for 15 minutes. While potatoes are roasting, mix orange juice and spices. After 15 minutes of roasting, add the bananas and spoon the spiced orange juice over the lot. Cook for an additional 10 minutes or so – until potatoes are tender and have browned. Bananas will soften and become striped (this is strange looking, but normal banana behavior). Remove to serving bowl and serve with just about anything, including your favorite holiday entrees.

NOT YOUR MOTHER'S WARM POTATO SALAD with MISO DRESSING (GF/V)

Roasted potatoes or other root veggies
olive oil
Sautéed deep greens (we used frozen chard from last summer)
Peas (frozen)
Sautéed mushrooms
Dressing of choice (optional)

Cut potatoes in chunks (probably around 1 ½ inches. Toss in a little olive oil, salt, paprika and pepper to taste. Roast in 450 oven on baking pan (single layer, spread out as much as possible) for about 25 minutes or until the outsides have browned and crisped and the insides are tender and heavenly.

To create our salad, I used the braised greens as a base, added a small pile of potatoes and added peas and mushrooms in my own personal pleasing ratio. Dressing is optional, but we found that this was delish with miso dressing. A creamier dressing or aioli would also pair beautifully with the potatoes.

Miso Dressing

1 Tbsp yellow miso (would likely work with other kinds, but I can speak with authority on the yellow)
1 Tbsp Bragg's or soy sauce
2 Tbsp rice vinegar
1 Tbsp sesame oil

Combine ingredients and whisk until smooth. This dressing is light in flavor and works well with both warm salads like the one above and more traditional fresh green salads.

OVEN COOKED ASPARAGUS (GF/V)

1 bunch of asparagus
1 Tbsp olive oil
salt and pepper to taste

Preheat the oven to 400. Wash the asparagus and cut off the woody ends. If your stalks are particularly thick, you may wish to peel them. Lay the asparagus out on a baking dish (I confess to having used foil on mine), keeping it in a single layer. Use a brush to coat the asparagus lightly with olive oil. Sprinkle with salt and a bit of pepper. Cover the pan with foil. Place in oven and cook for 10 minutes. Remove the pan, remove the foil and check the asparagus. Unless it's already cooked (unlikely, but if they're really small stems I suppose possible), leave the foil off and return to the oven for 5 more minutes. Check again and return to oven for no more than 5 additional minutes. The asparagus should be tender, but not limp or mushy.

PSYCHEDELIC SLAW w/ CARAWAY-MINT DRESSING (GF/V)
- adapted from the *Weight Watchers New Complete Cookbook*

6 Tbsp apple cider vinegar
3 Tbsp mayonnaise* (or whatever you use for that, I used a vegan substitute)
1- 1.5 Tbsp caraway seeds
1 Tbsp maple syrup
½ tsp salt
¼ - ½ tsp pepper
1 medium head purple cabbage
4 medium carrots
4 spring onions
4 Tbsp chopped fresh mint

Combine the first six ingredients in a bowl and whisk or stir with a fork and set aside. Shred the cabbage and the carrots (a food processor makes this a SUPER easy recipe). Chop the spring onions into whatever size works for you. Combine all the vegetation in a large bowl. Pour on dressing and toss.

SAVORY GREEN QUINOA (GF/V)

2 c quinoa
about 4 c water, divided
2 c spinach or other deep greens
½ tsp salt
Shake of nutritional yeast (opt)

Combine 2 c water and greens in blender and blitz the mess out of it. Add enough water to get 4 c liquid. Move the 4 c to a large saucepan. Add salt and bring to boil. While water is warming, rinse quinoa at least twice. When water boils, add quinoa, lower heat and cover. Cook for 15 minutes or until water is absorbed. Remove from heat and let it sit for 5 minutes. Fluff with fork. Add a shake of nutritional yeast if desired.

STRAWBERRY-SPINACH SALAD W/ BALSAMIC VINAIGRETTE (V)

Lots of spinach – torn or cut into the salad size you like
Fresh, luscious strawberries cut how you like
toasted pecans (dry warm pan, flip or stir periodically, take out of pan when you smell nuts- optional but awesome)

Throw in bowl. Toss. Done.

Vinaigrette

3 Tbsp olive oil, divided
1 Tbsp dijon mustard
1 Tbsp balsamic vinegar
salt to taste

Whisk together 1 Tbsp olive oil and the remaining ingredients. Whisk until fully incorporated and smooth. Set aside until is time to go to table. Add the last 2 Tbsp olive oil and whisk until smooth and delish.

STUFFED SWEET DUMPLING SQUASH (GF/V)

2 sweet dumpling squash (or other small round winter squash)
large handful dried apricots
handful of pepitas (or nut of your choosing)
much smaller handful of dried cranberries

1 ½ tsp olive oil
sprinkle salt and dried sage
Drizzle honey (optional)
little slip of butter (optional)

Preheat oven to 375. Oil a baking pan. Cut squash in half, scoop out the seeds. Level the bottom (not the scooped out side) so it will stay flat on the pan. Chop dried fruit. Mix fruit, nuts, olive oil and spices in bowl. Spoon into squash halves. Bake (stuffed side up please) for approximately 30-35 minutes.

Test your squash for doneness – it should be VERY easy to stick a fork in and pull some flesh away from the skin of the squash. Cooking times will vary according to the size of your squash. I did not add butter or honey to my own squash. Two of our tribe enjoyed theirs with a little melted butter.

SWEET & SPICY CARROTS (GF/V)

2 large carrots
1 tsp maple syrup
1 tsp cinnamon
1/8 tsp ginger
pinch of salt

Cut carrots into chunks and microwave for 90 – 120 seconds or to desired tenderness. Mix together remaining ingredients. Stir into carrots. Serve hot or cold. Make a double or triple batch and store in the fridge in little containers that can be grabbed – like a 'snack'!

THREE SLICE ROAST CABBAGE (GF/V)

1 head of cabbage
olive oil or oil of choice
salt and pepper
vinegar (optional)
other spices (optional)

Preheat oven to 400. One slice to cut the head in half and then 2 more to bring you to 4 pieces. Ain't math grand? I love it that 3 slices makes 4 pieces. Brush each quarter with oil of choice – I used olive, salt and pepper. Here is your first opportunity for variation. If you don't use much oil, or you would like to experiment with flavor, why not use sesame oil and a little soy sauce… or just a little soy sauce, or balsamic vinegar, or a little veggie broth, or some other sauce that you like. You could add herbs. Marjoram comes to mind… and of course oregano is always tasty on roasted vegetables.

After you've brushed, sprinkled or dumped, wrap each quarter in aluminum foil and place on a baking sheet. Bake at 400 degrees for 45 minutes to an hour and test for tenderness.

TWISTED RATATOUILLE prounounced rat-uh-too-ee (GF/V)

Oil for sauté
1 medium sweet onion – diced
1 medium eggplant – diced
1 28 oz. can of tomatoes (I used fire roasted)
½ tsp. tabil (see below)
1 tsp. harissa (in sauces section)
1 tsp. cinnamon
pinch of salt (optional)

Sauté the onion and tabil in oil until onions are translucent. Add eggplant and sauté until soft
Add tomatoes, harissa and cinnamon. Cook for another 10 minutes or so. Serve plain or over toasted bread or rice – or favorite grain.

Tabil:
from *Vegetarian Times*, June, 2013, p. 44:

¼ c coriander seeds
2 Tbsp cumin seeds
1 Tbsp caraway seeds
2 tsp red pepper flakes
2 tsp garlic powder

Toast all but the garlic powder in a small skillet – swirling constantly for about 3 minutes or until darkened and fragrant (and BOY is it fragrant), then transfer to a bowl. Add garlic powder, grind finely and store in an airtight container.

VEGAN CREAM BISCUITS (V)
– adapted from happyherbivore.com[96]

2 c whole wheat pastry flour
5 tsp baking powder
¼ tsp salt
4 Tbsp Not So Sour Cream (in sauces section)
2 Tbsp olive oil
1 c non-dairy milk

Preheat oven to 400. Stir together dry ingredients. Put in food processor, add NSSC and olive oil. Pulse until the clumps of creaminess and fat are not clumping. Return to bowl and stir in non-milk. Drop in ¼ c blobs onto greased baking sheet (or use parchment). Bake in oven on low rack for 15 minutes. Remove from oven and slather with whatever floats your biscuit boat. Try <u>Date Cream</u> (in breakfast section).

WHOLE WHEAT BOWTIES WITH ROASTED CAULIFLOWER (V Option)
- Inspired by Average Betty's Roasted Cauliflower[97]

1 batch roasted cauliflower (cut in pieces, toss with 1 tsp oil, bake at 425 for about 25 minutes – stirring at least once)
1 pound whole wheat bowties
1 Tbs olive oil
3 Tbs capers
1/3 c chopped fresh parsley
salt and pepper to taste
nutritional yeast or parmesan for garnish

As soon as cauliflower goes in the oven, set water on to boil for bowties. Assemble all other ingredients and place in large bowl. When cauliflower and bowties are done cooking. Add to bowl. Toss.

ZIPPY DAIRY FREE RICOTTA 'CHEESE' (or Teat-Free Ricotta) (GF/V)
- adapted from Little Sis' Nofredo Orzo with Chickpeas and Kale

1 c walnuts
2 T olive oil
2 T nutritional yeast flakes (opt.)
1 – 2 Tbsp rice wine vinegar (I accidentally put in 2 rather than 1 and I really liked the zip – try one and see what you think)
¼ c water
1 tsp salt
1.5 cup roasted cauliflower pieces
fresh ground pepper

Place all in the food processor and process. This comes out thicker than the nofredo sauce and is more like a ricotta or cottage cheese. If you want to make it thinner – add some water or non-dairy, unsweetened milk. Can be mixed with plain noodles, or with noodles or grains and veggies OR put a dollop on your traditional tomato based pasta dish.

ZUCCHINI-CARROT SLAW w/ CUMIN & LIME (GF/V)
- modified from *Weight Watchers New Complete Cookbook*

2 medium zucchini, grated (a food processor is easiest!)
4 carrots, grated
2 tsp ground cumin
4 Tbsp sunflower cheese (in dips section) mixed w/ 2Tbsp water (or sub mayo if you dairy)
1 tsp lime zest
2 Tbsp fresh lime juice
2 tsp chopped fresh cilantro
½ tsp salt
freshly ground pepper to taste

Using a food processor makes this dish take about 5 minutes. I think a hand grater would bump that up to 10. Julienne cut would take this up to about 25 minutes in my lazy estimation. Your call.

Add the cumin to next 6 ingredients. Whisk together. Pour onto zucchini and carrots. Toss to mix together. Chill.

Smoothies and Frozen Treats

CHOCONANA MILKSHAKE GOODNESS (GF/V)

2 cups whatever milky beverage floats your boat (I used a combo of coconut and almond)
2 Tbs chia seeds
2 frozen bananas, cut into pieces
1 Tbs raw cacao (I'm sure cocoa powder would also rock)
1 Tbs maple syrup

Put milk in blender with chia seeds to soak while peeling and cutting bananas. Add all remaining ingredients to blender and go to it! Makes 3 generous or 4 modest servings.

5 YEAR OLDS LOVE KALE SMOOTHIE (GF/V)

about 2 cups of kale leaves
2 bananas
about 1 peach worth of frozen peaches
fistful of frozen cherries
enough unsweetened almond milk to achieve blending

Mix in blender until desired texture is achieved. Add ice cubes if your team prefers a more frozen style smoothie. The cherries make it a bit brown rather than green, although when blending there was a moment when the top half inch was still pure green and it was deep pink below. I was tempted to stop and serve it right then, and next time I may do that very thing.

FOOD HANGOVER KALE SMOOTHIE (GF/V)

2 Tbsp chia seeds
1.5c water
2-3c fresh kale
2 frozen and 1 fresh banana
most of a can of pineapple and some of the juice
handful of frozen cherries
2 handfuls of fresh blueberries
1c cold water
handful of ice cubes

Place the chia seeds in a bowl or glass with 1.5c water and set aside. Place all other ingredients in blender. You may have more luck adding the items as you blend, depending on your blender. When you've finished assembling other ingredients, check chia seeds. They should seem a little jelly-like; if it's not, give it a few more minutes.

Baby Steps to Better Health / Recipes: Smoothies & Frozen Treats

Blend like mad and adjust ingredients to your preferences. My crew LOVED this one. I'm pretty sure we were close to the 3 cups of kale and the cherries added enough sweet and color to keep that reality from my children altogether. This made EXTREMELY generous portions for four very willing consumers. Delish.

HOMEMADE SPORTS DRINK (GF/V)

Mix the following in a small plastic container with a lid:

The Mix:
2 Tbsp Potassium chloride (salt substitute available at the grocery store)
1 Tbsp Sodium chloride (table salt)
1 Tbsp baking soda
1 Tbsp Cal-Mag (a powdered supplement of Calcium and Magnesium), or ground up calcium tablets

Quart sized jar
¼ tsp mix
½ - 1 c real fruit juice (i.e., contains just juice, not colored sugar water)
2-3 c water

Now you can make your mix simpler than this – I settled on this as a mix of different electrolytes because it helps us feel better after a heavy sweat, plus the name brands include potassium in theirs. You could just mix potassium chloride and sodium chloride if you wish. Or some recommend himalayan salt alone which has trace minerals in it. Just have your mix in your container handy.

I found another recipe that recommended using epsom salts (which are magnesium salt) in a sports drink and I have done so. Much cheaper than the Cal-Mag, but I only found that reference on 1 site and can no longer find it. You can skip the magnesium and calcium entirely if you want to.

Our little container lives on top of the fridge with a 1/4 tsp measuring spoon right beside it.

In a jar that is a little smaller than a quart I place 1/4 tsp of the mix and about 1/2 – 1 cup of natural fruit juice and fill it the rest of the way with water. This is less sugar than many recipes indicate, but hey, if you need carb replacing… eat a piece of fruit, or some other food rather than just adding more sugar to the drink.

Unless you are running marathons or seriously training and sweating, you probably don't need a whole lot of electrolyte replacing. *If you take blood thinners or diuretics, or have a heart condition, please consult your doctor before taking any potassium supplements or salts.*

ST. PATRICK'S SMOOTHIE (We Don't Need No Stinkin' Shamrock Shake) (GF/V)

Super creamy, super green, fantastic and delicious way to start a happy St. Paddy's Day. And not a pinch in sight.

2 c fresh pineapple
4 medium frozen bananas
4 c spinach or other deep greens
½ rolled oats
½ c unsweetened shredded coconut
2 c coconut milk
½ large avocado
1 Tbsp honey or maple syrup

If you have a power blender, load it up and let her rip as you usually do. If you have a standard blender, start with the milk and frozen bananas and add the other elements when possible.

TRICKY GREEN SMOOTHIE (GF/V)

2 cups squashed down kale
1 mango
2 & 1/2 frozen bananas
about 1/2 cup fresh pineapple
and enough unsweetened almond milk (or other milk) to make it go.

I made this one day when Little Sis was visiting with her (then) twin 5 year olds. I told the little people it was green because it was a 'green mango smoothie.' I even had a green-ish mango in the fruit bowl to demonstrate the green. After they had declared the smoothie delicious and were well past halfway, I allowed my (then) 11 year old to let them in on the other contributor of 'green-ness'. They continued drinking and professed delight in the concept despite having fussed previously over green smoothies that were too green in color. Ah yes, the things an Aunt can get away with.

Soups

AMERICAN BLACK BEAN SOUP (GF/V)
- adapted for speed and dairy considerations from Deborah Madison's Black Bean Soup in *Vegetarian Cooking for Everyone*

olive oil for the pot
2 c onion, chopped
1 c celery, chopped
1 c carrot, chopped small
2 c green pepper chopped small
4 bay leaves
4 tsp chopped rosemary
2 tsp dried thyme
2 Tbsp tomato paste
4 c black beans, soaked, cooked and drained or drained and rinsed from cans
4 quarts water
leftover grains if desired (I used 1.5 c cooked brown rice)
salt to taste
1 c Madeira
1 c coconut milk (or cream)
chopped parsley

Warm oil in the pot. Add onions and sauté for a few minutes. Add the rest of the veggies and herbs and cook until the color deepens a bit. Stir in the tomato paste and cook for an additional minute. Add the beans and the water. Bring to a boil. Lower heat and simmer, partially covered for at least 20 minutes. Add salt to taste and grains if using. Cook and additional 5 minutes.

Remove bay leaves and puree as much of the soup as your textural preferences dictate. A smoother puree can be achieved in a blender, but I don't like to do all that pouring of hot soup, so I use an immersion blender. Add Madeira and coconut milk (or cream if you do moo).
Serve with chopped parsley.

CARROT GINGER SOUP (GF/V)

3/4 cup cashew pieces soaked overnight in 1 cup water
5 c coarsely chopped carrots
1 c coarsely chopped onion
6 small garlic cloves – or a couple of big honkers (chopped)
1 tsp olive or other oil you prefer
1 tsp salt

Baby Steps to Better Health / Recipes: Soups

2 Tbsp grated fresh ginger (keeping ginger root in the freezer makes it easy to grate)
1 – 2 cups vegetable or chicken stock

After chopping veggies, sauté them in the oil until slightly tender and onions translucent. Add to high powered blender along with 1 cup stock, ginger and salt. Puree. Transfer to soup pot on stove to keep warm. Place cashews and water in blender (no need to wash blender) and puree on high until smooth and creamy. Add to soup pot and stir. Add more stock if desired to preferred consistency. Serve with bread or potatoes or crackers.

COLD KICKIN' SOUP (GF/V) (can help calm the symptoms of a cold – try it!)
- adapted from Ming Tsai's Immunity Soup[98]

1 Tbsp oil
1-2 jalapeños, minced with seeds
1 Tbsp minced fresh ginger
2 cloves of garlic minced
1 bunch scallions, green and white parts sliced
2/3 lb shiitakes, stems removed and tops 1/4-in sliced
2 ½ quarts vegetable stock
2 Tbsp soy sauce or Bragg's
about half a bunch of kale (I used a small mixing bowl full from the garden), torn from the big part of the stem, and ripped into manageable pieces
Juice and zest of 2 lemons
2 cups shredded carrots
Freshly cracked black pepper

Prep Notes: When chopping the jalapeño, I STRONGLY recommend wearing gloves, or putting plastic bags on your hands. This advice is particularly important for those of you who wear contact lenses. Yes, this is the voice of experience. OW. For the mushrooms, yes you really DO want to de-stem because the stems are quite rubbery. Most people who don't like shiitake mushrooms, don't like the stems. If you've got a microplane, use that bad boy to zest your lemons and your ginger.

Warm oil in a soup sized pot, just higher than medium. Add the jalapeño, ginger, and garlic. Sauté for about 2 minutes. Add mushrooms and scallions. Sauté for a few more minutes, being sure to give the mushrooms enough time to soften. Add your stock and soy sauce, bring to a gentle boil and cook for 5-10 minutes to allow the soup to reduce a bit and for flavors to mingle. Add kale, cook for about 2 minutes. Add lemon juice, zest, and carrots. Cook for two minutes longer. Add black pepper to taste.

COMPANY GOOD PEA SOUP WITH CRISPY LEEKS (GF/V)
- served four for dinner (with enough leftover for lunch for four) with bread and salad

olive oil for pan
1 leek
6 c veggie broth
5 c frozen peas
1 tsp salt
1/2 tsp ground pepper (I used white to hide it)
1tsp thyme
juice of 1/2 lemon
shelled fresh peas (I started with about 4 handfuls fresh, but you can just use however many you can get your hands on – or throw in some extra thawed frozen)

Let's start with the Crispy Leeks.

Cut the stiff green and the root end off the leek (save for future broth). Using the white and some of the light green part of the leek, cut the leek in half the long way and then in half again, you should have what looks like long pickle spears. Place the leek into a bowl of water and swish them around (leeks tend to hide dirt between the layers). Pour glug of olive oil into pan and warm on low. While oil is warming, remove leeks from water and cut into about 1/2 inch pieces (no, I didn't measure and never will, so there). Add leeks to pan. Proceed to largely neglect them for about 20 minutes, stirring periodically. This should be about how long you need to make the soup. They will begin to brown, and this is GOOD. Do not become alarmed. Reduce the heat a bit and keep an eye on them. You want to brown them as much as you can without burning them. If using cast iron, you can turn the pan off when you're getting close and just let them sit in the pan to finish up.

OK, so while your leeks are browning... The SOUP!!!
Pour half of the veggie broth in a blender. Add the frozen peas and go to it. If your blender doesn't like dealing with the frozen peas, add more of the broth. When blended, pour into a pot and add remaining broth, salt, pepper and thyme. Warm soup over medium heat (and don't forget to stir your leeks). When warm and your leeks are browned as you would like, add juice of 1/2 lemon. Stir.

Serve in bowls, adding a handful of fresh peas and a spoonful of crispy leeks. The fresh peas will barely cook (my limit on cooking for most fresh veggies) and will add just the right crisp bite to the velvety soup. Delish. That's company good.

CREAMED LENTIL SOUP WITH CELERY (GF/V)
– adapted from Dean Ornish's *Eat More, Weigh Less* version of the Deborah Madison recipe

1 onion, diced
1 c chopped celery
2 garlic cloves, smashed or minced
2 bay leaves
¼ c fresh parsley
1 ½ tsp salt
3 ½ c water
3 ½ c veggie stock
1-2 tsp Dijon mustard
2 tsp - 1 Tbsp red wine vinegar
pepper to taste
chopped celery leaves

Throw everything (gently) except the mustard, vinegar, pepper, and celery leaves right into a crock pot. Turn on high and allow to cook for about 4-5 hours. When you're ready to eat, puree in blender or use an immersion blender (I truly do love mine, no lie) to blend in the mustard and vinegar.

GINGERY SWEET POTATO BLACK BEAN SOUP (GF/V)

½ Tbsp coconut oil (or other oil you prefer)
1 medium sweet onion, diced
1 Tbsp. ground fresh or frozen ginger (freezing ginger makes it much easier to grate, although grated frozen looks like more than it is, so mash it down to measure)
1 tsp marjoram
5 cups chunked sweet potato (skin off or on)
juice 1 small lime
1 – 1 ½ tsp. chili powder
3 – 4 cups stock or broth
1 can coconut milk (I used light)
1 large apple, chopped (skin off or on) I used a pink lady
2 handfuls fresh baby spinach
2 cups cooked black beans (drained and rinsed if using canned)
Fresh cilantro for garnish (optional but yummy!!)
peanuts for garnish (also optional but also yummy!!)

Sauté the onions and ginger in the oil until translucent. Add chopped sweet potatoes, marjoram and chili powder and sauté for a few minutes. Add broth, coconut milk and apple. Bring to a slow boil and cook about 15 – 20 minutes until sweet potatoes are tender (will depend on how small you chunked). Smoosh the apples and sweet potatoes some. You could blend if you want, but I just smooshed, thickening some but leaving some bites and chunks. Add spinach and beans and cook a few more minutes to wilt spinach and heat up beans. Garnish with snips of cilantro leaves and peanuts.

LETOVER MASHED POTATO LEEK SOUP w/ WILTED SPINACH & BASIL (GF/V)

olive oil for the pot
1 leek, white and light green parts cleaned and chopped *
4 cups mashed potatoes
2 c water
½ tsp salt
fresh ground pepper
1 c coconut milk (or whatever you prefer)
olive oil for the pan
About 5 ounces of fresh spinach (or as much or little as you like – it DOES shrink a lot)
1 small clove garlic, minced or pressed
small handful of fresh basil, chopped

Warm olive oil in the bottom of a soup or stock pot, place chopped leeks and a sprinkle of salt in pot, sautéing and stirring occasionally until the leeks are tender and the white parts are a little translucent. Add the mashed potatoes and stir to combine. Add water and salt and stir to combine. Here's where we're gonna have some variation. If your mashed potatoes were perfectly cooked, had no lumps and were smooth as silk, you will only need to bring your pot of yum up to temp. If, like most of us, your potatoes were delicious but slightly less than perfect, you may want to bring the pot to a gentle boil to cook the potatoes just a little bit as the flavors mingle. When potatoes have reached the texture you prefer, add the coconut (or whatever) milk and ground pepper.

While the soup comes back up to temp, prepare the spinach. Warm olive oil to low-medium in a pan (I used cast iron). Add spinach, a sprinkle of salt, and the garlic to the pan. Turn/stir spinach frequently to encourage wilting throughout. When nearly all wilted, add the fresh basil. Stir for a little while longer. When all spinach is wilted and bright green, remove from heat. Serve soup with a few forkfuls of spinach, some lovely bread, and a salad.

* Leeks are dirty little suckers. When they grow up through the soil, they bring quite a bit with them, trapped in the layers. Cleaning them can be tricky. I simply cut the portion of the leek I intend to use into quarters the long way. I think place those quarters (they will separate – it's okay) into a bowl of water, let them sit while I prepare other bits, swish them around and then rinse. Works like a charm, every time, and I learned it at fancy cooking school, so it must be right, right? ;-) I can say that the bowl of water is always cloudy and dirty – so it seems to do the trick.

Baby Steps to Better Health / Recipes: Soups

LENTIL MINESTRONE (GF/V)
- Adapted from Deborah Madison in *Vegetarian Cooking for Everyone*

olive oil for the pan
1 ½ c chopped onion
2 Tbsp tomato paste (I freeze mine in a big blob on wax paper after I open a can and cut off what I need from the frozen blob)
2 Tbsp chopped parsley
4 cloves garlic
3 carrots cut small
1 c celery cut small
2 tsp salt
1 c lentils (I used green)
2 bay leaves, several branches parsley and a few thyme sprigs, (or dried herbs to taste)
9 c water or vegetable stock (I went halfsies)
Bragg's or soy sauce to taste
1 bunch greens, chopped (I used chard from the garden)
2 c cooked pasta (leftover works here as well)

Warm olive oil in a large pot. Sauté onion for about 10 minutes until soft and starting to brown. Add ingredients from tomato paste through the celery and salt. Cook for a few more minutes. Add the lentils, the herbs, and water/broth. Bring to a boil, lower the heat and simmer for about a half an hour. Taste and add salt and or pepper. Cook the pasta in a separate pot and drain. When the soup is ready, spoon pasta and raw greens into bowl and ladle soup on top. Add parmesan if that works for you. We dipped sunflower cheese bread.

LENTIL, MUSHROOM AND SWEET POTATO SOUP (GF/V)

olive oil for the pot
1 ½ c rough chopped onion
sprinkle salt
2 cloves rough cut garlic
2 cups thinly sliced mushrooms (I used cremini, but I think any mushroom would be lovely)
8 cups liquid (I used half veggie stock, and half water)
1 ½ c lentils (I mixed French and brown)
3 c cubed sweet potato
1 c chopped celery
2 Tbsp chopped fresh rosemary (or 2 tsp dried)
2 tsp minced fresh thyme (or 2/3 tsp thyme)
3 bay leaves
1 tsp smoked paprika

1 Tbsp Bragg's or soy sauce (opt)
2 c fresh tomatoes, rough cut (you could sub canned, but fresh is wonderful here)
¼ c red wine
loose chopped fresh greens of your choice

Warm the oil in a soup pot over low-medium heat. Add onions and a sprinkle of salt and allow to cook slowly until at least translucent. Add garlic and cook a short time longer. I let my onions go a good while as I did my chopping while they were cooking. I think this helps a lovely flavor to develop and recommend it if you have time. When onions are done to your liking, add mushrooms and continue to cook down a bit to let mushrooms release a little water. Add next 8 ingredients (all but tomatoes, greens, and wine). Bring to boil, reduce heat, cover and cook for at least 20 minutes. Flavor will develop with longer simmering, but lentils may "explode" if cooked too long at rolling boil. Watch your temp and test lentils for your personal lentil preference. When lentils have reached legume-y perfection, add tomatoes and wine. Stir and cook just a few minutes to warm. Serve over fresh greens in soup bowls and stir to wilt greens.

MI-SO-HONGRY….. ADAPTABLE MISO SOUP (GF/V)

Miso Broth

2-3 tsp miso paste per cup of water (I used 2 for a mild flavor)
However many cups of water you need to make enough soup.

Boil the water and then add the miso paste. The paste won't dissolve completely. If you've eaten miso soup in a restaurant, you've seen the same thing – thicker broth on the bottom, thinner broth on the top.

ADD-INs
While you're waiting for your water to boil, assemble your add-ins. If you want noodles, you should obviously start them first as well.

cooked rice noodles
thinly sliced mushrooms
shaved carrots
chopped cilantro
spinach
tofu

Others That Would Be Great

seaweed, of just about any kind
basil
lemon juice

red pepper
rice
spring onion

You really could put lots of things in there, and the fun of it for us was building that bowl of soup right at the table.   dished up broth for everyone and then we each constructed our own miso bowl, perfectly suited and seasoned for our taste preferences.

ROASTED BUTTERNUT SQUASH SOUP (GF/V)

2 butternut squash
2 onions
4 c of vegetable stock
1 cored but unpeeled apple (I used Gala), cut in half
½ - 1 tsp sage
1 tsp salt (or to taste)

Preheat oven to 375. Cut butternut squashes in half, scoop out the seeds. Peel and then cut 2 onions in half and brush them all lightly with your favorite oil. I brushed the bottoms of the onion and the tops of both. Place on a baking sheet and roast for about 45 minutes. I confess this is an estimate - you want the squash to be soft. This can be done ahead of time if you like. Let the squash cool to the point where you can pick it up, scoop out that gorgeous flesh and into a bowl for later use, or right into the high speed blender, or a pot where you can use an immersion blender. I do not have an immersion blender and have not tested this recipe, so user beware! I use a 14 year old Vita Mix. Place half of the ingredients in the blender at a time, mix til smooth and pour out into pot. Repeat and then heat, stirring occasionally.

SHWEET POTATO STEW (DF/V)
- adapted from Mark Bittman in The NY Times[99]

1 med – lge onion, chopped
oil for the pan
½ tsp chili powder
1 tsp fresh grated ginger (place fresh ginger in the freezer and it is very easy to grate with a grater or microplane.)
5 c cubed sweet potato (I left the peels on)
1 ½ c cubed apple (I also left the peels on)
1 c chopped carrot (I left the peels on….)
1 can light coconut milk
1 ½ c vegetable stock
fresh cilantro for garnish
peanuts (1 – 2 Tbsp per bowl) for garnish

Sauté onion and spices in pan until translucent. Add sweet potatoes, carrots and apple and cook for about 5 minutes. Add coconut milk and stock, cover and bring to a gentle boil. Cover and simmer until sweet potatoes and apples are very soft – about 20 minutes depending on how small your cubes of sweet potato are. Smush it some… or should I say Shmush it some with a masher. Serve garnished with cilantro and peanuts.

SLOW COOKER CREAMY TOMATO SOUP (GF/V)
inspired by – Savvy Vegetarian[100]

2 ½ c chickpeas
4 c water or bean broth*
2 Tbsp Bragg's or soy sauce
1 large can or box chopped tomatoes (or 6 ripe if in season)
2 bay leaves
1 tsp sugar (I used turbinado, but I imagine others would work just fine)
2 carrots, rough chopped
2 stalks of celery, rough chopped
2 cloves garlic, minced
1 tsp smoked paprika (you could sub out a VERY small bit of chipotle to get some smoky flavor without bite – similar strategy to my Smoky Baba Ghanoush)
1 tsp salt
2 Tbsp tomato paste
1 c milk (I used coconut milk)
chopped parsley (opt.)

This is an easy-peasy lemon squeezy dinner, friends. It is also easily adapted for the amount of time and effort that you are able to give it.

SUPER EASY APPROACH: Put everything but the milk in the slow cooker, turn it on low and cook for 6-7 hours. Puree with immersion or regular blender. Add coconut milk (or whatever you're using) and stir. Serve with parsley garnish (if you're fancy and like a little spring zing, which I am and I do).

SLIGHTLY MORE EFFORT: Sauté veggies in olive oil for a few minutes (5-10) before dumping in crock pot to give them a head start on softening. Add to slow cooker with all ingredients except for milk. Turn on low for 5 hours. Stir in milk. Garnish and serve.

VEGAN CURRY SOUP (or Not Just Kramer's Mulligatawny) (V)
– adapted from *The Best of America's Test Kitchen 2009*

serves 4-6, I always double, it freezes beautifully

2 ½ tsp garam masala
1 ½ tsp cumin
1 ½ tsp coriander
1 tsp turmeric
2 Tbsp coconut oil
1 ½ – 2 c chopped onions
½ c unsweetened coconut
4 cloves garlic, chopped
4 tsp minced fresh ginger
2 tsp tomato paste
¼ c wheat flour
7 c veggie broth or water
2 carrots, chopped
2 ribs celery, chopped
½ cup brown or French lentils, rinsed and picked through
salt and pepper
chopped cilantro for garnish
plain yogurt for serving (I used almond yogurt)
cooked brown rice for serving

Combine spices. Melt or warm coconut oil in large pot on low-med heat. Stir spices in and sauté until they smell awesome. Add onions and coconut and cook until soft (around 5 mins). Add garlic, ginger, and tomato paste and cook for another minute or so. Add flour and stir until ingredients are combined. Add broth and stir well, being sure to clean bottom of pan with the broth to get all of the spice. Add carrots and celery and bring to boil, lower heat and simmer for about 20 minutes (until carrots are soft). Puree however you like (I used a stick blender because I hate all of that pouring back and forth, but a blender will give you a cleaner puree and will do a better job on the coconut). Add lentils and bring to boil, reduce heat and simmer for 30-40 minutes. Salt and pepper to taste. We spoon rice into the bowl, add soup, a dolop of yogurt and a sprinkle of cilantro, but plain works too!

VEGETABLE, BEAN & BARLEY STEW (V)
– inspired by Barley Bean Vegetable Soup on Savvy Vegetarian[101].

1 ½ c garbanzo beans (canned or soaked and cooked)
1 ½ c navy beans (canned or soaked)
½ c pearl barley (soaked for at least 4 hours or cooked ahead of time)
6 c liquid from these sources: bean broth or soaking water, water, veggie broth (I used 4

Baby Steps to Better Health / Recipes: Soups

c bean broth and 2 c veggie broth)
2 Tbsp olive oil
2 med carrots, chopped to your preferred cooked carrot size
3 medium potatoes, peeled and cut to soup size chunks
4 leaves Chinese cabbage (this was my substitution for 2 stalks celery, which I'd run out of, the sub was successful)
2 cloves garlic, made very small however you prefer
1 tsp each: basil, thyme, oregano, smoked paprika (or regular paprika, I love the smoked paprika) ½ tsp ground fennel
1 bay leaf
1 Tbsp Bragg's or soy sauce
1 c frozen peas

As with many slow cooker recipes, there is still food prep to do, it just happens WAY in advance. For this particular recipe, the most frugal approach involves using dried beans. I started with one dry cup of each of the beans called for and soaked them in twice as much water in a pot overnight. This actually yielded more than the three cups total called for I think, but I threw them in anyway. If you like THICK soup/stew, you may want to do the same. I soaked the ½ c barley in a mason jar with water in the fridge overnight. Measuring these out the night before took me a total of about 3 minutes.

Drain the beans and barley. Set the beans in fresh water to boil (they were done in about 25 minutes, but times vary for beans). While beans cook, chop the veggies and then put the olive oil in a pan to warm. Add the carrots and cook for about 5 minutes. Add the potatoes, cabbage, and garlic. While the veggies are cooking, add the barley, the broth and all the spices to the slow cooker. Add the veggies and when the beans are done, drain and add them as well (saving the broth for future soups). Cook on low for about 4 hours. I believe it would be entirely reasonable to skip pre-cooking the veggies and put it all in the slow cooker for at least 6 hours. When we were ready to eat, add the cup of frozen peas and give it a good stir.

WILD RICE AND MUSHROOM SOUP (DF/V)
- adapted from *Moosewood Restaurant Daily Special* by The Moosewood Collective

1 c raw wild rice
3 c water
2 Tbsp olive oil
1 onion, chopped
1 c chopped carrots
1 c chopped celery
½ tsp dried rosemary
½ tsp dried thyme

2 bay leaves
2 tsp salt
3 c fresh mushrooms (the book suggests wild, I used cremini)
4 c water
3 Tbsp soy sauce
¼ c dry sherry
black pepper to taste

Bring rice and 3 c water to a boil in a covered pot. Reduce heat and simmer until rice is tender and water is absorbed – about 45 minutes. While the rice is cooking, heat oil in a large pot and sauté the onions for about 5 minutes. Add the veggies and seasonings and sauté for another 5 minutes. Stir in water, soy sauce and sherry and simmer for 10 minutes. Remove bay leaves. When rice is tender, stir into soup. Add pepper. We ate ours with some whole wheat bread and a green salad.

ENDNOTES

[1] http://www.youtube.com/watch?v=RV7Qz640OeM

[2] Shute, N., (2007). Over the limit? U.S. News & World Report, 4/23/2007, Vol. 142, Issue 14

[3] Sheridan, C., (2004). Private conference on Conscious Discipline. http://braintender.com/BT/conscious_discipline.html

[4] Dean, J., (2013). Making habits breaking habits: How to make changes that stick. Oneworld publications.

[5] http://www.sugarstacks.com/ Retrieved July 6, 2012

[6] Beil, L., (2013, June 1). Sweet confusion: Does high fructose corn syrup deserve such a bad rap? Science News, 183 (12), p23-25

[7] Beil, L., (2013, June 1). Sweet confusion: Does high fructose corn syrup deserve such a bad rap? Science News, 183 (12), p23-25

[8] http://www.heart.org/HEARTORG/GettingHealthy/NutritionCenter/HealthyDietGoals/Frequently-Asked-Questions-About-Sugar_UCM_306725_Article.jsp#.TxCSoltAF7M

[9] http://www.heart.org/HEARTORG/GettingHealthy/NutritionCenter/HealthyDietGoals/Frequently-Asked-Questions-About-Sugar_UCM_306725_Article.jsp#.TxCSoltAF7M

[10] http://www.heart.org/HEARTORG/GettingHealthy/NutritionCenter/HealthyDietGoals/Frequently-Asked-Questions-About-Sugar_UCM_306725_Article.jsp#.TxCSoltAF7M

[11] David Buchholz MD suggests a host of changes in diet to prevent migraines and MSG is on his list.
Buchholz, D., (2002). Heal your headache. Workman Publishing.
The Mayo Clinic also includes MSG on a list of foods to avoid for a possible connection to migraines.
Mayo Clinic, (2013). Migraine. http://www.mayoclinic.com/health/migraine-headache/DS00120/DSECTION=causes. Retrieved: September 1, 2013.

[12] Center for Science in the Public Interest, (2013). Chemical cuisine: Learn about food additives: Safety ratings key. Retrieved 8/11/13 from: http://www.cspinet.org/reports/chemcuisine.htm

[13] Moss, M., (2013). Salt, sugar, fat : How the food giants hooked us. New York : Random House.

[14] http://wholegrainscouncil.org/recipes/cooking-whole-grains

[15] Moss, M., (2013). Salt, sugar, fat : How the food giants hooked us. New York : Random House.

[16] Retrieved from University of Minnesota School of Public Health. Project EAT. February 4, 2012
http://www.sph.umn.edu/epi/research/eat/publications.asp#

[17] Eisenberg ME, Olson RE, Neumark Sztaincr D, Story M, Bearinger LH. Correlations between family meals and psychosocial well-being among adolescents. Archives of Pediatrics and Adolescent Medicine. 2004;158:792-796.
As cited by, University of Minnesota School of Public Health. Project EAT, Retrieved: February 4, 2012
http://www.sph.umn.edu/epi/research/eat/publications.asp#

[18] Eisenberg ME, Olson RE, Neumark-Sztainer D, Story M, Bearinger LH. Correlations between family meals and psychosocial well-being among adolescents. Archives of Pediatrics and Adolescent Medicine. 2004;158:792-796.
As cited by, University of Minnesota School of Public Health. Project EAT, Retrieved: February 4, 2012
http://www.sph.umn.edu/epi/research/eat/publications.asp#

[19] http://www.popsci.com/scitech/article/2006-05/science-confirms-obvious?page=3

[20] http://www.cbsnews.com/8301-504763_162-57369857-10391704/sugar-should-be-regulated-like-alcohol-tobacco-commentary-says/

[21] Sturt, J., (2011). Higher consumption of sugar-sweetened beverages is associated with increased risk of developing type 2 diabetes or metabolic syndrome. Evidence-Based Nursing, 14 (2), p. 35.

[22] http://www.care2.com/greenliving/ten-surprisingly-sugary-foods.html?page=10 Retrieved July 6, 2012

[23] http://www.sugarstacks.com/ Retrieved July 6, 2012

[24] WebMD, (2012). Retrieved February 8, 2012
http://www.webmd.com/diet/features/13-ways-to-fight-sugar-cravings?page=2

[25] Mayo Clinic, (2013). Nutrition and healthy eating: Which oil should I use for cooking? Retrieved September 3, 2013 from:
http://www.mayoclinic.com/health/cooking-oil/AN02199

[26] KU Medical Center, (2012). Integrative medicine: Healthy cooking oils. Retrieved September 3, 2013 from: http://www.kumc.edu/school-of-medicine/integrative-medicine/health-topics/healthy-cooking-oils.html

[27] KU Medical Center, (2012). Integrative medicine: Healthy cooking oils. Retrieved September 3, 2013 from: http://www.kumc.edu/school-of-medicine/integrative-medicine/health-topics/healthy-cooking-oils.html

[28] American Heart Association, (2013). Answers by heart: Lifestyle + risk reduction: High blood pressure: Why shoudl I limit sodium? Retrieved September 3, 2013 from: http://www.heart.org/idc/groups/heart-public/@wcm/@hcm/documents/downloadable/ucm_300625.pdf

[29] KFL&A Public Health (2007). Knocking out salt.
http://www.kflapublichealth.ca/Motiv8/Files/Knocking_out_salt.pdf

[30] Center for Science in the Public Interest, (2014). Chemical cuisine: Learn about food additives. Retrieved from: http://www.cspinet.org/reports/chemcuisine.htm

[31] http://www.cspinet.org/reports/chemcuisine.htm

[32] http://eatingmindfully.com/mindful-eating/

[33] "Whole foods are complex, containing a variety of the micronutrients your body needs — not just one. An orange, for example, provides vitamin C plus some beta carotene, calcium and other nutrients. A vitamin C supplement lacks these other micronutrients.
Essential fiber. Whole foods, such as whole grains, fruits, vegetables and legumes, provide dietary fiber. Most high-fiber foods are also packed with other essential

nutrients. Fiber, as part of a healthy diet, can help prevent certain diseases, such as type 2 diabetes and heart disease, and it can also help manage constipation.
Protective substances. Whole foods contain other substances important for good health. Fruits and vegetables, for example, contain naturally occurring substances called phytochemicals, which may help protect you against cancer, heart disease, diabetes and high blood pressure. Many are also good sources of antioxidants — substances that slow down oxidation, a natural process that leads to cell and tissue damage."
Mayo Clinic, (2013). Nutrition and healthy eating: Supplements, nutrition in a pill? Retrieved Nov., 7, 2013 from:
http://www.mayoclinic.com/health/supplements/NU00198

[34] Harvard School of Public Health, (2013). The nutrition source: What should I eat? : Health gains from whole grains. http://www.hsph.harvard.edu/nutritionsource/what-should-you-eat/health-gains-from-whole-grains/

[35] Sun Q, Spiegelman D, van Dam RM, et al. White rice, brown rice, and risk of type 2 diabetes in US men and women. Arch Intern Med. 2010; 170:961-969. As cited in: Harvard School of Public Health, (2013). The nutrition source: What should I eat? : Health gains from whole grains. http://www.hsph.harvard.edu/nutritionsource/what-should-you-eat/health-gains-from-whole-grains/

[36] Interesting article on this topic at The Center for Science in the Public Interest: https://www.cspinet.org/nah/articles/supersized.html

[37] NIH, (2013). National heart, lung, ad blood institute: Educational campaigns: We Can!(R): Eat right: Serving sizes and portions. Retrieved 11/14/13 from:
http://www.nhlbi.nih.gov/health/public/heart/obesity/wecan/eat-right/distortion.htm

[38] Dinner plate size has increased 23% from 1900. Wansink and Van Ittersum as cited in Arumugam, N., (January 26, 2012). How Size And Color Of Plates And Tablecloths Trick Us Into Eating Too Much. Forbes on-line: Lifestyle. Retrieved 11/14/13 from: http://www.forbes.com/sites/nadiaarumugam/2012/01/26/how-size-and-color-of-plates-and-tablecloths-trick-us-into-eating-too-much/

[39] Cal Dining, (2013). Serving size guide. Retrieved 11/14/13 from:
http://caldining.berkeley.edu/portion.html

[40] Carlson, A., & Frazão, E., (2012). USDA: Are healthy foods really more expensive? It depends on how you measure the price. Retrieved 01/12/14:
http://www.ers.usda.gov/media/600474/eib96_1_.pdf

[41] Nelson, J. K., & Zeratsky, K., (2012). Mayo Clinic: Nutrition and healthy eating: Nutrition-wise blog: A healthy diet is a smart investment. Retrieved 01/12/12 from: http://www.mayoclinic.com/health/cost-of-healthy-food/MY02252.

[42] CSA – Community Sponsored Agriculture, a sort of buy-ahead program for local farms whereby the consumer receives a set amount of vegetables per week at an agreed upon price based on seasonal availability. More information about this great way to eat fresh, local and healthy here: http://www.localharvest.org/csa/

[43] Everyday Choices, (2011). Fortify your health with a nutritious diet. Retrieved 01/15/14 from: http://www.everydaychoices.org/eat.html

[44] CDC, (2013). Diabetes public health resource: 2011 National diabetes fact sheet: Diagnosed and undiagnosed diabetes in the United States, all ages, 2010.

[45] American Diabetes Association, (2013). The Cost of Diabetes. Retrieved 01/15/14 from: http://www.diabetes.org/advocacy/news-events/cost-of-diabetes.html #sthash.1Y0WutUO.dpuf

[46] ADA, (2010). Diabetes Care: Diagnosis and Classification of Diabetes Mellitus. Retrieved from: http://www.ncbi.nlm.nih.gov/pmc/articles/PMC2797383/

[47] NIH, (2014). National heart, lung, blood institute: Clinical guidelines on the identification, evaluation, and treatment of overweight and obesity in adults: Executive summary: Summary of evidence-based recommendations. Retrieved 01/16/14 from: http://www.nhlbi.nih.gov/guidelines/obesity/sum_rec.htm

[48] ADA, (2014). Are you at risk? Retrieved 01/16/14 from: http://www.diabetes.org/are-you-at-risk/?loc=atrisk-slabnav

[49] McMullen, L., (2014). US News & World Report: Health: 7 reasons to choose a plant-based diet. Retrieved 01/16/14 from: http://health.usnews.com/health-news/slideshows/7-reasons-to-choose-a-plant-based-diet

[50] http://www.localharvest.org/csa/

[51] Whitman, W., (1900). *Leaves of grass*. Philadelphia: David McKay.

[52] http://www.merriam-webster.com/dictionary/nourishment

[53] http://www.merriam-webster.com/dictionary/nutriment

[54] American Heart Association, (2014). Circulation: Statement on xercise: Benefits and recommendations for physical activity programs for all Americans. Retrieved from: http://circ.ahajournals.org/content/94/4/857.full

[55] Johns Hopkins Medicine, (2014). Health library: Risks of physical inactivity. Retrieved from: http://www.hopkinsmedicine.org/healthlibrary/conditions/cardiovascular_diseases/risks_of_physical_inactivity_85,P00218/

[56] http://healingfeast.com/simple_changes.cfm

[57] http://acozyplacecalledhome.blogspot.com/2013/01/roasted-chili-lime-nuts-low-carb-gluten.html

[58] Madison, Deborah. *Vegetarian Cooking for Everyone*

[59] http://happyherbivore.com/2009/08/southern-style-biscuits-gravy/

[60] http://www.amazon.com/gp/product/1592334644/ref=as_li_ss_tl?ie=UTF8&camp=1789&creative=390957&creativeASIN=1592334644&linkCode=as2&tag=mysisspan-20

[61] http://www.gazingin.com/?s=sweet+potato+brownies

[62] http://detoxinista.com/2012/03/almond-flour-frosted-sugar-cookies/

[63] http://www.averagebetty.com/recipes/oatmeal-apple-muffins-recipe/

[64] http://whimsicaldesperation.wordpress.com/2012/08/24/buckwheat-chocolate-chip-cookies/

[65] http://www.amazon.com/gp/product/B004GKMI2S/ref=as_li_ss_tl?ie=UTF8&camp=1789&creative=390957&creativeASIN=B004GKMI2S&linkCode=as2&tag=mysisspan-20

[66] http://www.amazon.com/gp/product/B004GKMI2S/ref=as_li_ss_tl?ie=UTF8&camp=1789&creative=390957&creativeASIN=B004GKMI2S&linkCode=as2&tag=mysisspan-20

[67] http://voices.yahoo.com/vegan-chocolate-chip-cookies-1995179.html

[68] http://realfoodforlife.com/peanut-butter-bliss-balls/?awt_l=P2.es&awt_m=JHAJjguSJuvlTu

[69] http://www.tasteofbeirut.com/2011/05/oatmeal-and-chickpea-flour-cookies/

[70] http://gazingin.com/?s=sweet+potato+brownies

[71] http://www.gazingin.com/

[72] http://justblitherblather.wordpress.com/2014/02/12/collard-quiche-with-sweet-potato-crust/
[73] http://www.marksdailyapple.com/primal-paleo-pie-crust/#ixzz2PMYINdX3
[74] http://www.marthastewart.com/872940/cauliflower-steaks-roasted-pepper-and-tomato-salad
[75] http://www.vegetariantimes.com/recipe/chickpea-tikka-masala/
[76] http://www.vegetariantimes.com/recipe/chickpea-tikka-masala/
[77] http://goodcleanfood.wordpress.com/2012/06/02/thin-crust-sriracha-bbq-tofu-and-moxerella-pizza/
[78] http://ohsheglows.com/2012/10/05/glazed-lentil-walnut-apple-loaf-revisited/
[79] http://www.greenkitchenstories.com/mung-bean-stew-on-a-budget/
[80] http://littlehouseinthesuburbs.com/2008/11/perfect-pie-crust-step-by-step.html
[81] Isa Chandra Moskowitz's, Vegan with a Vengeance : Over 150 Delicious, Cheap, Animal-Free Recipes That Rock
[82] http://goodcleanfood.wordpress.com/2012/06/02/thin-crust-sriracha-bbq-tofu-and-moxerella-pizza/
[83] http://projects.washingtonpost.com/recipes/2010/08/04/spinach-chickpea-burgers/
[84] http://justblitherblather.wordpress.com/2014/02/12/collard-quiche-with-sweet-potato-crust/
[85] http://anunrefinedvegan.com/2013/01/22/smoky-chickpea-stew-with-spinach-sausage-cashew-cream/
[86] http://www.meatlessmonday.com/lemongrass-tofu-bahn-mi-sandwiches/
[87] http://www.meatlessmonday.com/recipes/tofu-au-vin/
[88] http://www.meatlessmonday.com/
[89] http://healthwithoutsacrifice.wordpress.com/2012/07/13/avocado-sauce-pasta/
[90] http://www.choosingraw.com/zucchini-marinara-and-the-power-of-friendship/
[91] http://mideastfood.about.com/od/dipsandsauces/r/harissa.htm
[92] http://emmycooks.com/2012/06/29/summer-berry-sauce/
[93] http://www.amazon.com/gp/product/B000VIMTYG/ref=as_li_ss_tl?ie=UTF8&camp=1789&creative=390957&creativeASIN=B000VIMTYG&linkCode=as2&tag=mysisspan-20
[94] http://ohsheglows.com/2010/02/23/glass-dharma-giveaway/
[95] http://www.mayoclinic.com/health/healthy-recipes/NU00566
[96] http://happyherbivore.com/2009/08/southern-style-biscuits-gravy/
[97] http://www.averagebetty.com/recipes/garlic-roasted-cauliflower-recipe/
[98] http://www.doctoroz.com/videos/shiitake-hot-and-sour-soup
[99] http://www.nytimes.com/recipes/12230/sweet-potato-stew.html
[100] http://www.savvyvegetarian.com/vegetarian-recipes/tomato-chickpea-soup.php
[101] http://www.savvyvegetarian.com/vegetarian-recipes/barley-bean-veggie-soup.php